Praise for *In Our Elem*

"When you're in your natural element you feel healthy, happy, and whole. In her book, *In Our Element*, Lindsay Fauntleroy...takes us on a step-by-step journey through the five elements of nature, Water, Wood, Fire, Earth, and Metal, and reminds us that we are not separate from nature; that nature is our mirror reflecting back to us our deepest needs. This book is medicine for the soul."

—Gail Parker, PhD, author of *Restorative Yoga for Ethnic and Race-Based Stress and Trauma* and *Transforming Ethnic and Race-Based Traumatic Stress with Yoga*

"Fauntleroy's scholarship is deeply embodied. It crosses continents, cultures, traditions, and centuries and is made all the more powerful by her personal and thoughtful reflections on our life and times...I highly recommend *In Our Element* for all who are inspired to seek, support, and integrate the healing both we and our world long for.

—Alaine D. Duncan, L.Ac., SEP, author of *The Tao of Trauma*

"An uplifting, sacred, and modern approach to ancient medicinal traditions and wisdom."

—Ashley River, author of *Tending to the Sacred* and *Messages from the Heart of the Divine*

"We live in a world where colonization and globalization have sought to erase the subtleties of who we are as people of color, and so many of us carry deep wounds that are ready to be healed. *In Our Element* is a book that will support our personal and collective healing as we co-create the future we have yet to boldly imagine.

—Aki Hirata Baker, Reiki master teacher and founder of MINKA Brooklyn

"*In Our Element* is a compelling, fun read! It is chock-full of practices and tools for self-awareness and discovery. Feast at Lindsay's banquet table of storytelling, interactive exercises, yoga poses, acupressure points, and flower essences for your favorite element!

—Katie Hess, author of *Flowerevolution* and founder of LotusWei floral apothecary

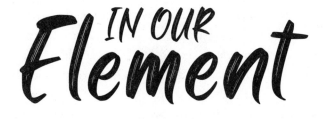

About the Author

Lindsay Fauntleroy is a medicine maker, educator, and acupuncturist. She was drawn to the healing arts after her own journey to fertility introduced her to the interconnectedness of body, mind, and spirit. Her clinical training includes a Master of Arts from New York University, a Master of Science from Tri-State College of Acupuncture, and clinical training in Traditional Chinese Medicine (TCM), Kiiko Matsumoto style Japanese acupuncture, and myofascial Trigger Point release. Lindsay is also a yoga instructor and a certified facilitator of Family Constellations Therapy. Her integrative approach to soul medicine integrates more than fifteen years of clinical practice with her doctoral studies of Indigenous and African Diasporic psychology.

Lindsay is passionate about the intersection of community wellness and social justice. Her school, The Spirit Seed, offers personal development workshops and practitioner trainings that honor Indigenous and African wisdom. Lindsay's Five Element-inspired flower essence remedies, the Elementals, are available in apothecaries and wellness clinics nationally and internationally.

Lindsay offers continuous gratitude for the lineage of ancestors, teachers, nature allies, and fellow neo-ancients who have supported *In Our Element*.

IN OUR
Element

• LINDSAY FAUNTLEROY L.Ac. •

Using the Five Elements
as Soul Medicine to Unleash Your
PERSONAL POWER

Llewellyn Publications
Woodbury, Minnesota

FIRST EDITION
First Printing, 2022

Book design by Colleen McLaren
Cover design by Shannon McKuhen
Interior art on pages 34, 47, 83, 134, 185, 231 by Llewellyn Art Department
Interior illustrations by Hollis Maloney

Llewellyn Publications is a registered trademark of Llewellyn Worldwide Ltd.

Library of Congress Cataloging-in-Publication Data (Pending)
ISBN: 978-0-7387-7054-3

Llewellyn Worldwide Ltd. does not participate in, endorse, or have any authority or responsibility concerning private business transactions between our authors and the public.

All mail addressed to the author is forwarded but the publisher cannot, unless specifically instructed by the author, give out an address or phone number.

Any internet references contained in this work are current at publication time, but the publisher cannot guarantee that a specific location will continue to be maintained. Please refer to the publisher's website for links to authors' websites and other sources.

Llewellyn Publications
A Division of Llewellyn Worldwide Ltd.
2143 Wooddale Drive
Woodbury, MN 55125-2989
www.llewellyn.com

Printed in the United States of America

Contents

Soul Medicine Practices

Quick Reference:
Summary of Soul Lessons

Water Element
Create an Oasis
Connect to the Source
You are Ancient

Wood Element
Anger = Change
Take a Stand
Express Yourself
Your Purpose has Power

Fire Element
You are Whole
Open your Heart
Joy has Juice
Your Senses are Sacred

Earth Element
Honor the Mothers
Find Your Center
Your Body is a Temple

Metal Element
Be Present
You are Precious
Let it Go

Disclaimer

The publisher and author assume no liability for any injuries caused to the reader that may result from the reader's use of content contained in this publication. Consulting with a trusted physical and mental healthcare practitioner is always recommended before beginning any exercise regimen or change in diet, and common sense is strongly urged when contemplating employment of the practices and substances described in this work.

Introduction

When you are in your element, you feel an amazing flow. You shine. You feel energized and vibrant. Your gifts and talents create abundance. You feel confident and authentic. Your relationships are loving and nourishing. You have a deep sense that you are fulfilling the deeper meaning and purpose of your life.

There are also times when you feel stuck. You may spend nights staring at the ceiling, filled with worry and anxiety. A weight of depression keeps you from enjoying the things that matter. You feel afraid, doubtful of your dreams, and unsure of the decisions that led you here. The point is there are times when you're in your flow, and times when you're not. This book will teach you how to align with the five elements to regain your footing, tap into your latent potential, and find your flow. I'll introduce you to the five elements—Water, Wood, Fire, Earth, and Metal—as a system for understanding our cycles and rhythms as part of a great and mysterious universal design. Each element has specific lessons, visible in the natural world. You'll learn how to recognize the signatures of the elements in the organic rhythms and cycles of your life.

True wellness includes tending to the hopes, dreams, desires, and frustrations of the soul. In this book, you'll learn to recognize "soul hiccups" such as heartache, confusion, anxiety, procrastination, depression, and more as signs that one of the elements wants attention. You'll also learn about soul medicine, which will immerse you in the wisdom and power of each element. Through self-reflection and each element's soul lessons, the healing magic of flower essences, embodied practices such as yoga and guided imagery, and music's cathartic force, you'll be empowered to rewire the thoughts and emotions that are short-circuiting your potential. They also help you to apply the ancient wisdom of each element to your life.

The five elements offer a blueprint for personal and collective transformation. Through a tapestry of rich cultural references and the intersection of spiritual traditions, I hope you find this ancient system still relevant in our tech-driven society. I share my personal experiences, as well as my insights from more than a decade of work with communities of color. I hope you will see that these vibrant, archetypal forces belong to *all* of us—and transcend race, class, gender, space, and time.

★★★

This book began writing itself almost forty years ago, when I was in elementary school. My best friend Lisa and I found a little shrub tree with a clearing on the inside with just enough space for two little girls to crawl into. There, we drew pictures in the ground with sticks and imagined ourselves to be ancient, conjuring witches. We believed wholeheartedly in the magic of the tree, and swapped stories of the secrets she whispered to us.

When I was twenty-three, by forces I still cannot explain to this day, I was the only woman traveling to West Africa with a crew of martial artists under the training of Heru Nekhet. As the menfolk went off to study, train, and do whatever menfolk do, I was left to my own devices. At one point, I sat under the wide, waxy leaves of a beautiful tree at the compound's gate. As I marveled at her intricate trunk of interconnected branches, a clear, distinct voice said, "You know I'm poison, right?" Her words of caution were cloaked in soft, sultry, and slightly seductive tones. But the funny thing is I didn't "hear" her with my ears. It was as if her voice directly entered my consciousness. Two minutes later, my teacher came outside and observed me marveling at the tree. "Watch out!" he exclaimed, alarmed. "That tree is poisonous!!!"

During that trip, I had the incredible honor of staying with the late priest Baba Ishangi, a renowned pioneer of African culture in America. Baba explained to me that if I wanted to harvest any herbs, I would first have to ask the Mother tree for permission. She governed the area and protected all growing plant life, and without her permission, the herbal medicine would not work. "Which tree is the mother tree?" I asked, eager to maximize my time and efficiency. "You'll know her when you find her," he explained. And off I went, looking for something but not having any idea what.

I did find her … or perhaps she found me. I know now she summoned me, as nature does when we open to her call. Since my tree fairy days, I've learned how to press my ear to her hollow and access nature's magic through my work.

This is how nature communicates with us. And this is the magic we are tapping into when we work with flower essences, soul medicine, and the five elements. This book is for those of us who want to reclaim a bit of the magic we've lost to our overly scheduled and technological lives.

A Bit about Me

I am a super nerd, and geek out about African and Indigenous medicine from all over the Diaspora. I am deeply committed to the healing arts and the cultures out of which they emerge. My research began in earnest with a master of arts from New York University, where I studied archetypes, myth, metaphor, and symbolism in media and popular culture. My graduate studies were heavily influenced by my work with African National Science (ANS), an organization that introduced me to the difference between the indigenous African and Western worldviews. My MA dissertation explored how materialism and individualism impact the psyche of communities of color.

My life changed drastically when I was diagnosed with premature ovarian failure in my midtwenties. I was devastated when my doctors told me that I was in active menopause and that I could never have children. This shattered the vision I had for my life, which included returning to the Gambia with my seven children in tow. My sister-in-law, Karen, had what seemed like hundreds of flower essence remedies in her kitchen cabinet. After listening to me bemoan my fate and heartache for hours, she carefully selected one of the bottles and shared it with me. The flower essences were a game changer! Not only did my heart finally find some peace, I also began to attract the right situations, people, and opportunities needed for my transformation. I spent more than two years fully committed to healing my body with natural medicine. This included my first acupuncture treatment with my mother-in-love, Shadidi Kinsey.

Dr. Kinsey began her studies under Dr. Mutulu Shakur at the Harlem Institute of Acupuncture. She was also my first acupuncture teacher. On her shelf was an old, crumbling book called *A Barefoot Doctor's Manual*. The barefoot doctors were working-class folks, who were trained in the basics of acupuncture and herbal medicine. These healers brought the medicine into rural and poor communities, where the highly trained wealthy doctors would not go. This has greatly influenced my own approach to this medicine—I believe it belongs to all of us, and that we should have access.

The deep immersion in the spiritual and healing arts while I was trying to conceive awakened my attention to synchronicity and meaningful coincidences. I studied intensely at an African spiritual organization, the Ausar Auset Society, where I was first introduced to the system of the five elements through qigong practices for emotional balance. Dreamwork, meditation, prayer, and ritual became the guideposts on my journey, illuminating the interconnection between my body and spirit. I used movement practices to release the stress held in my womb, and experienced the direct effect my emotional state and unresolved trauma had on my physical health. The spiritual work within this supported community ultimately led to the birth of my vibrant, healthy daughter.

My journey left me so enamored with acupuncture and spirituality that I read every book I could find before ultimately deciding to go back to school for a master of science in acupuncture. At Tri-State College of Acupuncture, I studied Traditional Chinese Medicine (TCM), Kiiko Matsumoto-style Japanese acupuncture, and myofascial Trigger Point release. In school, I earned the nickname "Trauma Mama" because of my interest in the intersection of personal crisis, emotional distress, spirituality, and the five elements. I knew I was on the right path when I began to study Alchemical Acupuncture under friend and colleague Lorie Dechar, who introduced me to the psychological and spiritual aspects of acupuncture theory.

As an acupuncturist, I have used the five elements as the foundation for courses in leadership, abundance, relationships and entrepreneurship. My curriculum for middle- and high-school students has been implemented in New York City public schools, and teaches urban youth how to work with music, meditation, and the five elements for emotional self-awareness and academic success. In fact, many of the music selections you find in this book were suggestions from my students, whose fingers are on the pulse of a changing world. Though ancient, the five elements are alive and well. This book is born out of years of personal practice, along with researching, teaching, and helping others to tap into the five elements as potent forces of healing.

I've found a home away from home in my treatment room and in healing circles, holding space for women as they move through their trauma and create entirely new lives for themselves. I've supported hundreds of women as they discover how to truly live in their element. Some of the women were, like me, trying to find a way to heal their bodies despite their doctors' ominous diagnoses. Others were vying for top positions in their companies. Others were trying to birth babies, books, or businesses. Others were on the front lines as activists for social change. And others were simply trying to piece their lives back together after heartache. My experiences have taught me an ancestral truth: There is no healing of the body that does not include healing the soul and spirit. And there is no healing of the soul and spirit that does not include nature.

I live in two worlds: I have a Western mind and an African heart. I believe in magic, I believe in science. My goal is for the resources that I share with you in this book to be both practical and magical. I hope that you will use them, that you will experience incredible shifts as you tap into your greatness, and that you will pass on these resources to support your family, friends, clients, and community. There is a lot of soul healing work to be done out there. And I'm glad that we are in this together.

About the Elements

There are some disciplines of Chinese Medicine that help us find our constitutional element. Though this book is about the five elements, it's a different approach than other Five Element or acupuncture theory books you may have picked up. The goal is not to determine your personality type or your destined health challenges as a fixed reality. You are not an element—you are *all* of the elements.

In my experience, my life has flowed through different phases, and each phase has amplified a different element within myself. I've been so Fiery that people have mistaken me for an extrovert, and nestled so quietly under my rock that people have mistaken me for a recluse. In an independent Wood phase of my life, I traveled solo to Jamaica and Paris. I worked a little too hard to prove myself at a high-end fashion brand. I also went through an intense eight-year Metal phase, when I devoted myself with nun-like austerity to initiation in priestess training in an African spiritual system. There, I learned divination, herbs, crystals, astrology, and the system of the five elements. As you'll learn, each element has a signature stamp on the ways we experience and navigate our life circumstances.

Each of the five elements lives and breathes within us, showing up in different junction points and inviting us to step fully into our power, our soul's calling, and our destiny. This book was written to teach us how to tap into those currents. The system I am sharing is ancient, originated by Taoists in the shamanic Xia dynasty (ca. 2205–1766 BCE) and Shang Yin dynasty (ca. 1700–1050 BCE). One theory states that the founders of the Xia and Shang dynasties came from the Fertile Crescent via present-day Iran, carrying with them shamanic spiritual practices that have ancestral roots in Nubia.[1] The system of the elements was cultivated and preserved throughout the Zhang dynasty all the way through the Communist Revolution, when it was stripped of many of its spiritual underpinnings. The Five Element system now lives in the Western world wearing the names of Chinese Medicine, Acupuncture and Oriental Medicine (AOM), or simply Eastern Medicine.

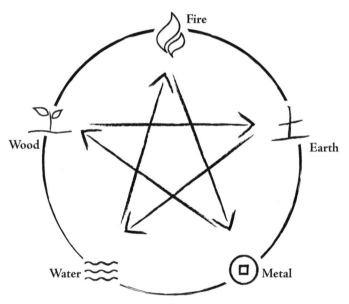

Five Elements Wheel

---

1. Clyde Winters, *The Ancient Black Civilizations of Asia* (Chicago: Uthman dan Fodio Institute, 2015).

Water—The Seed
Season: Winter
Phase: Incubation, seed of potential
Energetic: Down, sinking
Gifts: Introversion, intuition, reflection, stillness, caution
Emotion: Fear
Color: Blue/Black
Sound: Groaning

Wood—The Sprout
Season: Spring
Phase: Beginning, initiation
Energetic: Upward
Gifts: Self-actualization, purpose, vision, growth
Emotion: Anger, righteous indignation
Color: Green
Sound: Shouting

Fire—The Flower
Season: Summer
Phase: Blossoming
Energetic: Outward, expansive
Gifts: Extroversion, joy, relationships, love
Emotion: Love, joy
Color: Red
Sound: Laughing

Earth—The Fruit
Season: Late summer
Phase: Transition, change
Energetic: Spinning
Gifts: Nurturance, family, community, manifestation
Emotion: Empathy, overthinking
Color: Yellow
Sound: Singing

Metal—The Leaves
Season: Fall
Phase: Death, decline
Energetic: Dissipating
Gifts: Transformation, alchemy, the present moment, discernment
Emotion: Grief
Color: White
Sound: Sighing

Now you might be thinking, "Oh, I have lots of fire in my birth chart." Or, "I'm an earth sign." You're referring to astrology, another ancient, archetypal system. In fact, all ancient systems have a connection to nature. Indigenous traditions, African Diasporic Orisa systems, ayurveda, and the chakra system—to name just a precious few—are all nature-based psychologies with their own systems of element associations. However, each of these systems best keep their integrity when explored on their own, without trying to remix them together. Think of it this way: fire is fire is fire. But fire represents something different to the person who lives in Antarctica than it represents to someone living in the desert. So even though fire is fire is fire, for now, *this* Fire is not *that* Fire. *This* Water is not *that* Water. But at the same time, none of the systems are wrong. You are invited to think yes/and, instead of either/or. Resist the urge to be an element colonist, imposing your understanding of an element on another person or culture. Please and thank you.

Wu xing is the term most often translated as the five elements, but its true literal translation is the "five changes." In oracle bone script—the earliest known form of Chinese writing—the character *xing* is "the image of an intersection and symbolizes the connection of all energies and all directions."[2] Water, Wood, Fire, Earth, and Metal represent five movements, stages, and transformations. They represent the stages of visioning and manifesting your heart's desires, and the organic life cycle in which all things are conceived, birthed, expanded, and ultimately die. The five elements are a guide and a system for organizing all that we experience as the manifestations of a greater

---

2. Master Zhongwian Wu, "Daoist Imagery and Internal Alchemy," in *Transformative Imagery: Cultivating the Imagination for Healing, Change and Growth*, ed. Leslie Davenport (London: Jessica Kingsley Publishers, 2016), 196–212, 198.

universal pattern. Whether you find this to be scary or exciting, tapping into the flow of these five currents offesr us a great potential for change. You can work with these energies to create the life you want.

What Is Soul Medicine?

Take a minute, right now where you're sitting, to think about the healthiest person you know.

Go ahead, I'll wait.

Got it?

Awesome. Now for the next thirty seconds, write down all the words you would use to describe this person.

★★★

I've posed this question nearly a hundred times over the past ten years of leading workshops and retreats. And you know what? No one has EVER described the healthiest person they know as "free from a particular disease." Ironically, sometimes the opposite can be true: the healthiest person we know might be battling cancer or struggling with a degenerative disease like lupus or multiple sclerosis. And sure, you may have thought of a person who inspires you with their dietary regimen and exercise game. But most likely, the person who came to your mind is healthy because of *how* they move through their life—not because of their physical body.

Maybe they are positive and upbeat, and make you feel better about your own life just from being around them. My friend Keiana is like that. I swear it doesn't matter what the hell I tell her, she will always empower me with some affirmation that helps me see that my life is unfolding as it should. She has the unique ability to find the good in every situation without being annoying about it.

Maybe the person you thought of can approach whatever you throw at them with an air of calm and composure. My friend Trena is like that. I remember doing a walkthrough with her as she prepared for a high-stakes event. She had single-handedly organized a conference, which invited over thirty-five hundred students from all over New York City together for performances and workshops. Community politicians and stakeholders all had their eyes on her. In the moments before showtime, I was practically having an anxiety attack at the sheer enormity of it all. But Trena didn't break a sweat. She redirected every crisis thrown at her as if she were directing planes on a runway. Needless to say, the event was an incredible success and one of the highlights of her career.

Maybe the person seems to have it all together. Their parenting, their career, and their love life all seem to flow. My friend Lurie is like that. She manages to host a radio show, raise a baby and a teenager, and be kind and loving to her husband, all while having her hair and nails done. I thought her trade-off was in domesticity, but nope! One day I came over for dinner and found her making zucchini noodles. From scratch. Did I mention she's also an attorney? And that she finds time to respond to my random texts about *way* less important things, like the exact shade of brown of my new boo? I get heart palpitations as I consider her daily to-do list.

We all know amazing people who laugh often, have a positive outlook, and move through the world with grace and ease. The point is we know that true health is not just about how we feel in our physical bodies but also how we feel inside of ourselves. The healthiest people we know are tapped in to something that is beyond just physical health and material success.

Soul Medicine Is about Energy

Soul medicine is any medicine that helps us heal the subtle, intangible aspects of our being that are necessary to feel healthy, happy, and whole. There are plenty of resources out there to get physically healthy, but this book is about that sumthin' sumthin' that makes our lives flow. And that something has a name: qi. Qi is the animating life force that makes everything move, from our thoughts and feelings, to our bones and muscles. Qi is what makes some people feel like they're giving off good vibes, and why we feel "at home" in certain places. Qi is what makes us suddenly stiffen when someone walks a little too closely into our personal space, and it is what makes us melt into the arms of a lover. Qi makes plants grow and seasons change. Qi is an invisible current of energy. It is everywhere, all of the time.

Qi flows like a river. When a river gets blocked with debris, you get a buildup of too much stuff on one side of the blockage. Swamped with gunk, things get mushy, stagnant, and overwhelmed. On the other side of the debris, there's not enough water. Things on that side of the blockage wilt and die from the dryness and heat. Nothing can really thrive until that debris gets removed and the river can flow smoothly. That pretty much sums up the whole science of acupuncture, as far as I'm concerned. Acupuncturists use those tiny needles to clear the body's qi rivers, called meridians. Then, every organ and cell can get the qi flow it needs.

When qi is flowing properly, we experience good physical health. When qi is not flowing smoothly, we experience pain, inflammation, and disease. But that river can get blocked in any aspect of our life, not just our body. We can feel stagnant and blocked in our relationships, our finances, our creativity, our parenting, our career, etc. Over the years, I have found that my clients are drawn to soul medicine to harmonize their qi in one (or more!) of the following areas: money, honey, or health.

Money: Money is not just about financial abundance. When our "money qi" is flowing, we are able to live 'on purpose' and discover ways to bring our gifts and talents into the world. We experience abundance and prosperity in the form of resources, time, love, children or accomplishment.

Honey: Healthy "honey qi" brings pleasure and sweetness to our experience. It includes self-love and appreciation, connection to a spiritual sources, and a sense of loving kindness in our most important relationships. When our "honey" is right, we enjoy our lives and feel a sense of connection.

Health: As we'll discuss throughout this book, health is not just physical. Good health also includes mental clarity—knowing what to do and when to do it. We have the vitality to experience the joy of being alive, as well as emotional self-awareness and equanimity.

How to Use This Book

Books proudly line several shelves in my office, my bedroom, and my living room. Books about spirituality. Books about medicine and healing. Books about politics. Books about being Black. Books about being a woman. Books about being a Black woman. Books about love. Books about parenting. Books about business. Self-help books from every perspective. My books are like old friends, and each reveals a bit about me, what I care about, and what I think about most.

Here's the thing. I have not read a single one of these books on my shelf from cover to cover. Not a one. I am notorious for not finishing books—even books that I adore. I read a bit, highlight this and that, skip chapters, write notes in margins, and put them right back on the shelf. Sometimes I pick them up again and I am drawn to chapters that I had no interest in reading the first time around.

I wrote this book with the expectation that you will also jump around a bit and take it off the shelf when it calls. *In Our Element* is meant to be like a friend you call when you get stuck. It's for when you feel out of your flow, want to get back on track, and need a lil' energetic push to break through to the other side. This book isn't meant to be about theory, even though I personally find the theories of ancient medicine absolutely fascinating. This book is meant to be about *practice*—how you can embody this ancient wisdom and use it to transform your life.

There are a few ways to approach the material in this book. You can browse through the table of contents or leaf through the pages and trust what you feel drawn to. You may be picking up this book for the first, third, or thousandth time and know exactly which element to explore. Maybe you've been working with an acupuncturist, and you want to enhance the treatments you've been getting with some lifestyle changes. You can also review each element as a primer at the start of each season. Trust yourself, get in where you fit in, and enjoy the discovery!

There are hundreds of ways to work with the elements to create mind, body, soul, and spirit wellness rituals that work for you. I'd like to introduce a few allies for exploring, living and aligning with the elements on your path to personal discovery and transformation. I encourage you to personalize this process: pick and choose what works for you, and expect that even that may change over time. In this book, I'm offering a few menu selections that have served me well. Think of these practices as soul first aid: they are affordable, easy, and you can do them anywhere. In each chapter of the elements you'll find:

+ soul lessons and soul medicine practices;
+ flower essences;
+ embodied practices with yoga, visualization, and affirmation; and
+ "Music is Medicine" playlists.

Soul Lessons and Soul Medicine Practices

Each element teaches specific soul lessons modeled by nature to help us rewire our faulty mental, emotional, and spiritual programming. A great metaphor for the mind is an iceberg. The tip of the iceberg that peeks above the water represents our conscious mind: all that we can actively perceive with our five senses at any given time. The rest of the iceberg—beneath the water—is the stuff we *don't* know. That stuff is running amok with its own agenda and generally wreaking havoc in our lives. It's the parts of ourselves we can't see, the fears we didn't know we have, and the dreams we can't remember that hold the precious keys to unlock our greatness. That iceberg under the water is the home of our nervous system, our instincts, and our reactivity. Our inner dialogue goes something like this:

> "I'm gonna get up early to meditate every day this week! Let me set my alarm for 5:30 a.m."
>
> (Inner Wild One): *hits snooze three times so that I wake up twenty-seven minutes late and no longer have time to meditate*
>
> "I feel terrible when I eat sugar and dairy. I'm going to eliminate them from my diet." *pats self on back
>
> (Inner Wild One): *"Beesh! I am tired and stressed out so I'm gonna get some goddamn Haagen-Dazs before I lose my shit!"* *eats entire container of Rum Raisin*
>
> "I want to be in a committed relationship. I love this man and think he will make a great partner. I'm going to lean in and make this work."
>
> (Inner Wild One): *"He just did that thing that reminds me of the last guy who broke my heart! I **cannot** go through that again! Abort mission and shut the heart down, STAT!"*

My point is that our lives work best when our conscious self and our Inner Wild One are on the same page, working toward the same goal. Because nine times out of ten, the Inner Wild One is gonna take the reins. The tools in this book offer a way to get to know the Inner Wild One, instead of trying to ignore and silence them. They, like the elements, are a force of nature.

The journal prompts and soul medicine practices in each chapter will help you enter into loving conversation with your Inner Wild One. It may be helpful to keep a journal that you use specifically for your personal insights into the soul lessons of each element.

Flower Essences

I swear, flower essences are nature's best-kept secret. Flower essence remedies have been around for thousands of years—we even find symbolic carvings of flower recipes on the walls of ancient Egyptian structures. They were reintroduced as an alternative medicine in the West in the 1930s, which means we're looking at nearing a hundred years of this medicine being commercially available. I've been practicing this medicine professionally as a certified practitioner since 2009. In 2015, *Vogue* magazine featured an article on flower essences in which they were described as the "new Prozac."[3] In late 2016, Gwyneth Paltrow featured an interview with a flower essence practitioner on her lifestyle and wellness blog, *GOOP*. Yet, that doesn't stop even the people closest to me from asking, "Can I put your flower essences in my diffuser? How do they smell?"

The first thing you should know is that flower essences are not the same as essential oils used in aromatherapy. Flower essences have no scent, and putting them in a diffuser will do absolutely nothing but make your room smell like brandy (which is what's used to preserve them). Flower essences are a natural medicine to support energetic healing, and they work their magic when taken internally as herbal supplements. For those who are sensitive to alcohol, many companies make flower essences that are preserved with glycerin or apple cider vinegar. Adding flower essences to a cup of hot water will evaporate all traces of alcohol, or you can mist flower essences in your room or sacred spaces.

One of my colleagues describes flower essences as "vitamins for the soul." For those of you who have ever dabbled with weed, ayahuasca, or mushrooms, you know firsthand how plants can affect our consciousness. Flower essences are safer and more accessible, and offer hundreds of ways of thinking and feeling. If you've never dabbled with any of the other substances, think about the subtle shift you felt the last time you went on a nature walk, saw a

---

3. Eviana Hartman, "Are Flower Essences the New Prozac? Inside Fashion's Far-Out Healing Craze," *Vogue*, February 4, 2016.

beautiful piece of art, heard music that touched your soul, or were inspired by an unexpected message from a friend.

Flower essences are tools for increasing our self-awareness. They bring our attention to limiting beliefs that are under our radar, emotions that are out of control, and distorted perceptions that are blocking our success. Flower essences introduce us to the higher truths of our souls, offer healing for our heartache, and respond to our confusion and challenges with wisdom. Taken over time, they can create shifts at the soul level that result in unexpected miracles in our outer lives. They are nature's allies who remind us what it means to be truly human—the substance of this earth and the spirit of the stars.

In the fields of herbalism and plant medicine, every plant has an intelligence. It has a knowing, a higher truth, for us that it shares with humanity. Nature has been here for millions of years. Sometimes I think about the trees in Brooklyn looking down on us and thinking, "Oh, these humans … if they only knew X, Y, and Z." These trees have survived wars, floods, and the best and worst of humanity. This is why Indigenous psychology—practiced by medicine men, women, and shamans—has always integrated plants into healing rituals.

For each element, we'll explore my favorite flower essences, along with the soul hiccups that cut us off from our fullest potential. Each flower essence offers its own wisdom—a quiet mind, a patient heart, clear intuition, etc. You'll learn how to welcome this plant intelligence into your home medicine cabinet. Out of thousands of flower essence remedies, the ones I introduce in this book are my tried and true favorites. You can easily find these in specialty health food stores or online. See the recommended resources section at the end of the book for more information on where you can find flower essence products.

Here are some quick tips about flower essences at a glance:

+ Flower essences work hand in hand with self-awareness: they help us process difficult emotions, shift our perspective, and reprogram limiting beliefs.
+ Flower essences are not essential oils—they are usually taken internally and do not have a scent.
+ Flower essences are registered in the United States as dietary supplements.

+ The standard dose is four drops under the tongue, four times daily or as needed for stress.
+ Work with one flower essence or one flower essence formula for a minimum of two weeks, but ideally at least four weeks.
+ Flower essences are subtle yet profound—be mindful, journal, and pay attention.

Flower essences work through resonance, and so they are simply amplifying virtues and qualities that already exist within you. It's like turning up the volume on one instrument so that you can hear it more clearly and distinctly within the symphony. The more mindful you can be of your thoughts, emotions, and actions, the more effect you will notice. As you work with the flower essences in this book, stay on the lookout for:

+ vivid, revealing dreams;
+ a sudden "Aha!" moment—an affirmation or a statement of higher truth that comes to the surface to replace a negative thought;
+ a solution that previously evaded you;
+ deeper insight into your behavior or feelings;
+ relationship dynamics that shift as others notice, celebrate, or even resist your transformation;
+ new reactions to challenging situations; and
+ synchronicity—unexpected opportunities or new "chance" connections that propel you toward your goals or offer deeper insights.

Flower essences help us to pay attention to, turn off, or reprogram the inner dialogue of limiting beliefs that keeps us from reaching our goals, as well as facilitate a change in perspective. As we begin to see the world differently, the world around us begins to change.

Embodied Practice: Yoga, Visualization, and Affirmation

The meridians of Chinese Medicine are channels of energy that flow like rivers. These meridians circulate the energy, consciousness, intelligence, and wisdom of each element through our bodies, in the same way that the blood vessels bring blood to each organ and cell. Together we'll explore where these meridians fall on the human body, as well as key yoga poses that activate those channels. If you are new to yoga, you may feel something shift by simply bringing your attention to those places where you are holding tension or experiencing pain. If you are an experienced yoga student or teacher, you can layer these asanas, visualizations, and affirmations into your sequences as you explore the themes related to each element.

In Chinese Medicine, there are three kinds of qi in the universe: Heavenly Qi (*shen*), Earthly Qi, and Human Qi (*ren*). We, as humans, stand between the forces of Heaven and Earth. Three is a sacred number—it represents a totality of being. For example, we think of time in terms of past, present, and future. Holistic wellness considers body, mind, and soul. In the principles of inner alchemy, this trinity is known as the Three Treasures: Jing, Qi, and Shen. Daoist Master Zhongwian Wu explains:

> We consider Jing, Qi and Shen to be the best medicine in the world. *Jing* means essences and represents our physical body and Earth…*Qi* means vital energy and is related to our breath and energetic body and to all living things. *Shen* means spirit, and is your spiritual body, higher consciousness, and also represents Heaven. No matter what traditional art we are practicing, we always work with these three Great Medicines.[4]

The Three Treasures are incorporated into the embodied practices:

Jing: the actual physical alignment and position of your body in the suggested yoga postures

Qi: bringing awareness to your breath, and the emotional currents you will access as you breathe into the meridians of each element

Shen: the visualization, mental picture, and affirmation that accompanies each posture

Rather than completing a full yoga sequence, I invite you to explore the poses one at a time as you work with the soul lessons for each element. Cultivating awareness of the Three Treasures will help bring the gifts of that element more clearly into your life. You are welcome to explore these exercises

---

4. Master Wu, "Daoist Imagery and Internal Alchemy," 196–212.

as a formal seated meditation, a five-minute morning quickie, or anything in between.

Music Is Medicine

One of the most powerful ways we can experience the five elements is through music. Most of us have had the experience of using music as medicine. Maybe we have a playlist that we play for our workout to push us to the finish line. There might be a song that always cheers us up no matter what. There are songs that make me want to cry each and every time I hear them, no matter what is going on in my life. Certain songs remind me of home, of love, of love lost. Some songs bring inspiration. Some songs make me want to have hot, passionate sex. If you've ever seen someone catch the holy ghost dancing to house music, then you probably understand the song "Last Night a DJ Saved My Life."

I have used music as healing medicine throughout my entire life. Songs of the 1980s and 1990s retell the story of my childhood and coming of age. However, I learned just how powerful the integration of music and yoga could be when I discovered Sacred Yoga studio in Brooklyn. Though I had been practicing hot yoga for ten years, the classes at Sacred felt especially magical. And then I realized—it was the music! My favorite teachers knew how to time the chorus of the right song to hit at just the right time, during a difficult peak pose, or to invite the body to surrender at the end of practice. My experience in class inspired me to attend the Transformation class of Sacred's yoga teacher training in Costa Rica. Our teachers, Dara and Stephanie, had our class compile a collective playlist of our favorite songs with the theme "transformation," and the music carried us through the intense fifteen-hour days of yoga practice and study. Now, as a yoga teacher, I put just as much intention into the playlist my for classes as I put into the sequence of poses. Though Sacred sadly closed their doors in 2021, they left a legacy of incredible teachers who use music as medicine.

Music can shift our qi, and act as a tuning fork for any of the five elements that needs a little boost. Here's an example. One day I was running incredibly late for post-grad acupuncture training, for which I was the only Black student enrolled. Now, if you're Black, you might already intimately know the culturally imposed shame and taboo of being late for *anything* professional. But I had a three-year-old, which means my morning no longer belonged entirely to me. So, I was already in my feelings as I got on the train, threatened by a locked and loaded inner voice of "*see … this is why you shouldn't be. … This is why you can't. … blah, blah, blah.*" Instead of entertaining that voice, I put on my "Wood Element: Bawse Bitch" playlist and rocked out for the forty-five minutes of my train ride.

I got to the training an hour late with another student looking equally disheveled and chagrined. When we entered the classroom, the teacher (clearly taking our tardiness as a sign of disrespect) announced, "Well, since you two are so late, one of you might as well go back downstairs and get me a coffee."

Now, that people-pleasing-straight-A inner child in me would have said "yaaas missus" in her most subservient voice and gone scurrying to fetch that latte with her tail between her legs. But I, my true self, had been listening to my "Wood Element: Bawse Bitch" playlist, and feeling the self-assured righteousness of the Wood element. So instead, I pulled out a five-dollar bill for my partner in crime and sweetly smiled, "while you're down there, can you get me a latte too?" Then I graciously took my seat on my throne—I mean desk—and got down to work. It was a Good Wood day.

Each of the five elements corresponds with a sound, or a movement of energy. As you get to know each element, you'll also get to know the specific way they move your nervous system and the emotions they evoke. You'll begin to recognize their sounds, in yourself, your family, your friends, your lovers, your neighbors, the lady ringing up your groceries, etc. In each chapter, I'll introduce a playlist of contemporary hip-hop, rock, and R&B songs that capture the energy and emotion of that element—but this is just a starting point! I must warn you that my coming of age was in the nineties, and most (if not all) of my inspiration comes from the golden era of hip-hop. I encourage you to create your own music and medicine playlists as you explore the elements in your life. I hope that you will add to these playlists and make them your own.

★★★

The soul medicine we'll explore in this book helps us to look at our relationships, our careers, our bodies, our *everything* with a whole new mind. And that, my dears, is how we begin to transform our lives. That is how we live in our element. Because, as Albert Einstein once said, "No problem can be solved from the same level of consciousness that created it."[5] Or as my mama says, "If you always do what you always did, you'll always get what you always got." Or as I like to say, "Been there, done that!"

5. Gary Parker and Albert Einstein, *400 of Albert Einstein's Best Quotes: A Reference Book* (Self-published, 2021), 34.

Chapter 1
Changing Our Lens

The dictionary defines a miracle as "an effect or extraordinary event in the physical world that surpasses all known human or natural powers and is ascribed to a supernatural cause."[6] What I've learned in my years of practice is that we are *all* capable of experiencing miracles, and our miracles show up in many ways:

The miracle of loving again after your husband dies in a tragic accident

The miracle of finding the courage to walk away from a lucrative corporate job to launch your dream business

The miracle support that shows up to help you leave that not quite abusive, yet not quite heathy relationship

The miracle of finding an affordable apartment in Bed-Stuy, Brooklyn, against all odds

The miracle of running into an old friend that gives you just the right insight at just the right time

The truth is we are surrounded by miracles. They are, quite literally, everywhere and happening all the time. The problem is we can't witness miracles with our regular eyes and ears. By design or by default, our senses are simply not made to process the incredible shifts that happen in the subtle space between the mind and body. In order to experience miracles, we need a new lens, one that is able to see to the level of the soul. This chapter introduces a

---

6. "Miracle Definition & Meaning," Dictionary.com, accessed October 18, 2021, https://www.dictionary.com/browse/miracle.

few concepts that help adjust our lens, so that we can understand how soul medicine works. These foundational concepts are:

+ yin and yang theory,
+ the four states of consciousness, and
+ the subtle body.

Yin and Yang Theory

We can't fully understand the five elements until we understand a concept that is central to Five Element theory: yin and yang. These two forces of darkness and light, the moon and the sun, represent the most ancient of archetypal energies. This psychology of yin and yang shows up in many ancient cultures, though with different names. In the hieroglyphics of the pyramids, we find representations of two deities called Shu and Tefnut, personifications of the forces of light and darkness, expansion and contraction. In Dahomey mythology of the Fon peoples of West Africa, the deities Mawu and Lisa represent the sun and moon, respectively. In the Ifa tradition, one of the oldest surviving religions, patterns of alternating light and dark comprise the Odu Ifa, a divination system that gives insight into energetic currents underlying our experiences. Similarly, the *I Ching* divination system of Chinese culture and philosophy is based on patterns of alternating yin and yang. As with the Odu Ifa, this pattern of light and dark is represented by single (yang) and double (yin) lines. Fast forward a couple thousand years, and we find this binary pattern in coding, the foundation of computer science and digital technology. Just like in the movie *The Matrix*, this light/dark on/off polarity can create entire worlds. Yin and yang are the basis of everything, a natural fluctuation between light and darkness that is the language of the universe, holding the keys to the kingdom.

According to the Daoist cosmology, the primordial state of our universe consisted only of one swirling mass of qi. Within this mass, there were two different qualities of qi: (yin qi (heavy, turbid, and chaotic) and yang qi (light, clear, pure). After a very long time, all of tin qi Settled downward and formed the earth, while all yang qi rose upward to form Heaven.[7]

---

7. Master Wu, "Daoist Imagery and Internal Alchemy," 196–212, 200.

Yang is considered the Divine Masculine, and the yin is considered the Sacred Feminine. However, this concept is not related to earthly gender or physical form—the terms describe how qi moves. From this perspective, no matter how we identify in our physical body or gender expression, we all have both yin and yang qi within us. These two concepts are not opposites but instead complements. Together as an integrated whole, they teach us about the oneness of life. Just as you can't have a coin with only one side, and just as the daytime defines the night, yin and yang represent a continuum of two dynamic, interrelated forces that depend on each other for existence. The following table summarizes the qualities associated with yin and yang:

YIN	YANG
Moon	Sun
Dark	Light
Cold	Hot
Heavy	Light
Hidden	Revealed
Intuition	Intellect
Introversion	Extroversion
Body	Mind
Soul	Spirit
Stillness	Activity
Slow	Fast
Sacred Feminine	Divine Masculine

Yang is associated with the sun and the Fire element, which are about movement and expansion. It is expressed in things that are hot, dry, and move quickly. In North America, the summer is the most yang time of year—the sun shines bright for long hours, it's hot outside, and everyone is ready to party! Here in Brooklyn, summer kicks off with Dance Africa!, a colorful, festive marketplace and festival known as much for its social sightings as it is for its renowned dance performances. This joyous event embodies the yang energetic.

The yang is light, both in the sense of being weightless, as well as in the sense of being bright and revealed. We can see things clearly. Our thoughts, perceptions, and mental activity are yang in nature. The spiritual gifts of yang energy include awareness, revelation, and enlightenment.

At the other end of the spectrum we find yin, which is associated with the moon and the Water element. Yin is about substance. Whereas yang causes things to expand, things that are yin contract into themselves. Yin is dominant in things that are cold, wet, and move slowly. Winter is the most yin time of year. Imagine a cold, snowy day, when you just want to cuddle up under a thick, heavy blanket with tea. Yin brings us deep within ourselves into quiet and stillness. It has a hidden nature, similar to how the plant and animal world retreats underground for the cold months. Rather than energy and dynamic movement, yin relates to the substance of our physical body, nature, and our earthly experiences. Our emotions, our body's knowing that evades conscious awareness, and our subconscious mind are all yin in nature.

In a perfect world, yin and yang are balanced, equally represented and equally valued. But as we know, we do not live in a perfect world. The modern, technological society we live in is what I call "yang dominant," one in which yin and her associated qualities are still struggling for equal R-E-S-P-E-C-T. In this patriarchal society, the masculine (yang) has an advantage, as evidenced by the predominance of men gaining larger salaries and more opportunities than their women-identifying colleagues.[8]

In addition, the qualities associated with yang—logic, reason, rational thought, and productivity—get more props than emotions, feelings, and relaxation. We also associate the forces of light with goodness, and forces of darkness with evil. The beauty and wellness sector is a multitrillion dollar industry that celebrates youth and longevity (yang), while devaluing the beauty and wisdom that is part of aging (yin). Our smartphones and Amazon Prime subscriptions cater to our desire for instant access (yang), and we get frustrated and impatient when things move slowly and take a long time (yin). The dominance of yang over yin is also reflected in how we treat our bodies. When we say things like "mind over matter," we affirm that we value what we think more

---

8. Lois Frankel, *Nice Girls Don't Get the Corner Office: Unconscious Mistakes Women Make That Sabotage Their Careers*, (New York: Grand Central Publishing, 2014).

than what our body is experiencing or feeling at any given moment. Nature, including our bodies, is something to be conquered. This schism in the Western psyche was used to justify race-based slavery and the annihilation of Indigenous communities, and dismiss spiritual practices steeped in the mystery of nature and the unknown.

When it comes to working with soul medicine, there are two important things to know about yin (well, actually there are about a thousand things to know, but these two are really important): (1) yin moves slowly, and (2) timing is everything.

1. The Yin Moves Slowly

Yin and yang are a team, and they work together like a happy couple. Yang sets or affirms our attention in the mental realm, while yin gives things concrete actions and form in the physical world. We can't create anything in our lives without these two forces working harmoniously. Here's a concrete example. Imagine I want to go on an amazing tropical vacation. The yang part of me can immediately envision the sandy beach, the cool waters, myself in a skimpy bikini, lying in a hammock with a frozen piña colada. Yang moves fast—before you even finished reading that sentence, I was there … and maybe you saw yourself there too! The most yang aspects of our being are our intention and imagination, and they move faster than the speed of light.

Next on the spectrum of yang to yin comes our emotions. After I get the mental image of my hot sexiness on the beach, I start to feel excitement and anticipation. Mixed in there are feelings of peace and relaxation as the sun sets in my mind's eye. Yup, it feels good! In the continuum of yang to yin, our feelings and emotions are more yin than our thoughts and ideas. That means our feelings change *after* our thoughts and perceptions.

For me to manifest this vision and to actually get to this beach, I've got to attend to the details of the earth. That means checking my calendar, booking a plane ticket, and packing the luggage. It's going to take some time for all of those pieces to come together. Yang is free from time and space—I can be anywhere instantly in my mind. But my body, the substance of me, can only be in one place at one time.

Which is right now sitting on a chair in front of my computer writing this book.

When we are working with soul medicine, the yang moves faster than the yin, which means that our thoughts and perceptions are going to change first. Our feelings are going to change next, though a bit more slowly than our ideas and mental images. And our physical circumstances (our body, job, relationships, money, etc.) are going to change last. Each shift is valuable but if we are not mindful, we will miss the subtle changes in our thinking and feeling, psyche and soul, that happen before the big changes in our lives are evident.

2. Timing Is Everything

I grew up in a time and place where girls were taught that just kissing a boy could get you pregnant. Believe it or not, there is a whole generation of forty-something-year-olds who avoided public toilets because of the pregnancy risk. You can imagine my surprise when it took me nearly two years of earnest trying and a few suspiciously spent nights upside down to get pregnant. But I digress. In Yin and Yang theory, the sperm represents the yang. As long as they are healthy, those fast lil' swimmers can create life anytime and anyplace (cue Janet Jackson). But the yin, the egg, is bound to laws of time and space. The egg has a narrow window of fertility. In some women, the open window for the egg to receive the sperm lasts about twelve hours. In other women, that window is only an hour or two. Whatever it is, it is very specific. Those little swimmers hit the egg at the wrong time and guess what? Ain't nothing happening. The egg waves to the sperm, "Sorry, try again next month!" through a window slammed shut.

Timing is everything. When a woman gives birth, she surrenders to timing that cannot be controlled. I had an elaborate birth plan for my daughter, but she came much more quickly than I expected. Do you think it would have been possible for me to say, "Hold on little baby, you can't come until I set up my meditation room?" Nope! Her destiny was to be born at a specific time, and there was nothing I could have done differently. I often share my story about my nephew, who was born at 24 weeks and weighing only 1.25 pounds. When his parents say that he was born early, I remind them: He came at the exact right time. You guys got pregnant late! The timing of the yin is connected to destiny—and it's nonnegotiable.

To create what we desire, our intention (yang) needs to align with the substantive power of the yin. Our intentions and imagination are without limits, but it takes time for life on Earth to catch up with the images in our mind. Yin welcomes us into her dark mystery through the tools that help us align with divine timing—astrology, divination, dreams, delays and obstructions, or a good friend who gives you a reality check. Yin is the energetic force that allows us to respect and tap into the divine timing of our unfolding lives.

States of Consciousness

In modern tech-based societies (yang-dominated) we tend to value logos over eros. *Logos* is a Greek word that refers to the principle of judgement and reason, the root of the word "logic," while *eros* is Greek word related to feeling and passion (the root of the word "erotic"). We think people are intelligent when they have a strong command of language and the ability to articulate clearly while speaking or writing. They figure out things quickly, while their yin-oriented comrades take a longer time to "feel their way through" things. In this culture, we don't necessarily call people intelligent when they are intuitive or emotionally saavy. If anything, emotional people are called "irrational" or "emotional" (as if those are bad things!). The word "lunatic" is a not-so-subtle diss, with the Latin word *luna*, or moon, at its root.

In addition to our intellect, our brains have access to different states of awareness and perception. These are measured by the speed of brain activity in cycles per second, measured in hertz (Hz). These states of awareness lie on a continuum from most rapid (yang) to those that move slowly (yin).

Beta State (13-40 Hz): Awake, Logical, Responsive

The beta state is our most yang state of awareness and is designed to help us function in the physical world. In a yang-dominated society, it makes sense that this state of awareness is the most common and familiar. Beta is an active and alert state in which we can consciously process information received from any of the five senses. The beta state is also the home of our rational, linear, and logical thinking. It's the area of the brain we use to calculate, strategize, process information, and analyze the world around us.

As you are reading this book, you are likely in a beta state of making sense of the words on the page and determining if it aligns with your personal beliefs and experiences. It's a heightened alertness that we use when we're walking across the street in New York City, making sure there are no cars coming. In a beta state, we can do things that require our full attention—take an exam, play sports, give a presentation, analyze and organize information, and other activities where mental alertness and high levels of concentration are essential to success.

Alpha State (7-12 Hz): Contemplative, Energetic, Emotional

As brain activity slows down and becomes more yin, we move into the alpha state. The alpha state of awareness and perception is a place of easy relaxation just below our conscious awareness. As you are reading this book, every now and then you might slip off into a daydream or memory. Or maybe you start to drift off into thoughts about what you are going to make for dinner. We move in and out of the alpha state of awareness fluidly throughout the day as we shift from active, conscious thinking into soft space and time. Have you ever had the experience of getting home but not remembering how you actually got there? You don't remember passing certain landmarks. You don't remember swiping your Metro card or driving past the grocery store. You were on autopilot. That's the alpha state.

The alpha state is a light meditative state of passive visualization, creativity, and imagination. We can purposefully come into the alpha state for creative solutions through practices such as meditation and deep breathing. In alpha awareness, our imagination, visualization, memory, and concentration are expanded. In this state, we can also perceive the energetic movement of qi in response to emotions—a knot in our throat, butterflies in our stomach, love radiating in our chest. The alpha state is one of the most effective states of awareness to perceive the energetic currents of the five elements.

Theta State (4-7 Hz): Associative, Dreamlike, Symbolic

The theta state is even more yin than the alpha state; we have to slow down quite a bit to get there. Theta awareness and perception opens the REM dream state and intuition. This is a place of deep meditation and heightened receptivity, where insight appears as nonverbal flashes of dreamlike images. It is a highly symbolic state, and deeply connected to archetypal symbols and their associated meanings. In the theta state, we can perceive the shape of a lion forming in the clouds, or the image of two people arguing in a blot of ink. One of my dearest friends enters the theta state to decipher images and meaning from coffee grounds during Assyrian rituals and ceremonies, an Indigenous tradition that she has passed on to her daughter. The theta state of our awareness projects and perceives symbols and images as messages for the soul.

In addition to dreams and meditation, we can access this state through hypnotherapy, active imagination, guided imagery, divination, and dreamwork. Flower essences are thought to interact with the theta state by ushering subconscious material into conscious awareness. This is why flower essences often elicit vivid dreams or an attraction to stories or characters. Our theta mind is also activated when we strongly resonate with a myth or character. Divination systems such as tarot or astrology rely heavily on our ability to relate to archetypal symbols and images and can facilitate tremendous life shifts through our theta state of consciousness.

Delta State (0-3 Hz): Sleep, Trance, Unified Consciousness

If we keep going down, down, down into the depths, we come to the delta state of awareness. The delta state is the most yin state known to modern science; it is a deep stillness, like the bottom of the ocean. We access our delta awareness in the kind of deep, restorative sleep where we wake up with drool in the corner of our mouth, not quite sure what day it is. During the delta state, human growth hormone is released, making this stage of sleep important for healing and replenishment. Delta awareness is also transpersonal—it connects us to worlds beyond our own. In addition to sleep, this state is induced by certain African and Indigenous rhythms to connect to universal consciousness. Meditation and chanting are also portals to the delta state.

We better understand the five elements when we greet them through our alpha, theta, and even delta states of awareness. These states also help us to perceive the subtle yet profound shifts that happen when we work with soul medicine. If we look through the lens of only our logical and rational minds, we miss most of the magic.

The Subtle Body

Beta consciousness grounds us in the physical world, which we perceive with our five senses. But just because we cannot see, taste, hear, feel, or touch something, it doesn't mean that it isn't real. There's a spectrum of energy that our eyes can perceive: red, orange, yellow, green, blue, indigo, and violet. In the Western world, we learn to name the colors of the rainbow—ROY G. BIV— at an early age. Naming the colors somehow makes them more real than our actual wonder and experience of them. But we also know that infrared light and ultraviolet light exist outside the spectrum of what our eyes can perceive. If we didn't believe in something we couldn't see with our own eyes, we wouldn't have gel manicures or wear sunblock. In this day and age, it would be almost crazy to say that infrared or ultraviolet light don't exist because we can't see them. The same science is at play with a dog whistle. The dog hears it, but we don't. That because dogs' ears can perceive a different spectrum of sound waves than our ears. But it would be silly to say that there's no sound just because we can't hear it. Our five senses were designed to only perceive a specific range of frequencies, but there is so much more out there. And the same is true of the physical body.

There is an aspect of our body that extends beyond the material, which the ancients called the subtle body. The subtle body has many different names but is consistently present in Indigenous and Diasporic healing systems.

The Physical Body

When we talk about health, the physical body is usually what we're talking about. The physical plane relates to any aspect ourselves that we can see, taste, touch, hear, or smell. The physical body is substance—bones, flesh, muscles, organs, blood, and cells—making it the most yin aspect of our being. We experience our physical bodies through the beta state of consciousness.

Healing in the physical body requires either biochemical and biomechanical change. Biomechanical healing modalities that address the physical plane include surgery, physical therapy, and any kind of exercise program that manipulates the body's actual physical structures. Biochemical modalities include food as nutrition—achieving optimal health through balancing vitamins, minerals, and the micronutrients necessary for good health. Healing on the physical plane also includes pharmaceutical drugs, which directly affect the neurotransmitters in the brain, the mechanical processes of the organs, or other chemicals in the blood.

In a medicine based on the science of the physical plane, specialization in medicine allows the body to be separated into parts that can be studied and addressed, unfortunately in some cases without the consideration of how these parts may affect the whole. Luckily, we can upgrade our physical health regimen by integrating complementary and alternative modalities that target the subtle body.

The Etheric Body

Modern science is starting to come around to a truth the ancients knew: everything has a frequency. When we move beyond what we can readily perceive with the five senses, the first plane we come to is the etheric body. Also called the emotional body, the etheric body can be described as an energetic field that envelops the body's physical structures. This energy is neither biomechanical nor biochemical but instead electromagnetic. In order to perceive this aspect of the subtle body, we have to leave our beta state of awareness and enter into the realm of alpha consciousness.

The etheric plane is experienced as movement of energetic pulses. It relates to the natural vital force of the nature, prana or qi. This life force exists in both humans and nature, so medicines for the etheric plane restore the proper flow of life force as reflected in nature. Practices include breathwork, gemstone and crystal therapy, or simply finding peace in solitude in nature. The etheric plane is also strongly connected to our emotions, the natural expressions of life force that create harmony or disharmony in our life experience. Music is an incredibly effective medicine for the etheric plane. Beyond the lyrics, melody and rhythm have the capacity to lift and expand our spirits or collapse us into sadness. Music moves the life force.

Plant medicines that resonate with the etheric plane include herbs and essential oils, which are often classified in their respective materia medicas by their influence on the movement or direction of the life force. Chinese Medicine is a system strongly tied to the etheric plane. The legend tells us that acupuncture itself emerged from the practices of an ancient shaman who drove stakes into pressure points on the earth to bring down the rains. Similarly, acupuncture needles are placed in the pressure points of the body (a metaphor for the earth) to regulate energetic flow. Whether this story is true or myth (or both), it reminds us that we humans are energetically connected to the earth.

The Astral Body

We access the next layer of the subtle body, the astral body, through our theta state of awareness. The word "astral" has the Greek root word *astra*, also found in *astronomy* and *astrology*. Indeed, the astral plane relates to "light" energy, or the energy of the stars. The astral body is also known as the mental body, and it relates to our thinking and beliefs, and the filter through which we interpret our experiences. The astral body encompasses the constellations of beliefs and perceptions that are the foundation of our personality.

Changing our thoughts and perceptions has tremendous healing power. In his book, *You Are the Placebo: Making Your Mind Matter*, Dr. Joe Dispenza explains:

> We see our beliefs as truths, not as ideas we can change. If we have very strong beliefs about something, evidence to the contrary could be sitting right in front of us, but we may not see it because what we perceive in entirely different. We've in fact conditioned ourselves to believe all sorts of things that aren't necessarily true, and many of these things are having a negative impact on our health and happiness.[9]

Our astral body responds to myths, stories, and symbols that help us understand the mysteries of the universe. Here, imaginative images come to life.

In the astral body, healing comes from accessing the thoughts, perceptions, and interpretations of our experience. In other words, let's change the narrative! Healing modalities include talk therapy, counseling, and meditation. Creative visualization and working with affirmations help us to replace limiting beliefs and ideas with those that are life-affirming, thereby moving us more assuredly toward our goals. In divination systems such as Ifa, the Babalawo[10]

---

9. Joe Dispenza, *You Are the Placebo: Making Your Mind Matter* (Hay House, Inc., 2015), 166.

10. *Babalawo* is the name for a chief priest in the Ifa spiritual systems.

will cast the Odu Ifa.[11] Within the reading there will be stories, medicine and wisdom that will properly align a person with the correct flow of their destiny. A skilled astrol ger can give insight into the perceptions and personal myths that resonate with a person's attitudes and perceptions. This brings healing at the level of the astral body as a person realigns with their cosmos. In other instances, a movie, a myth, or even a character in a book creates a resonance with the astral body that allows us to shift our perspective and find healing in our life story.

Finally, flower essences are one of the most effective plant medicines for facilitating healing at the level of the astral body. They work directly on our thoughts, change our perceptions, and shift the limiting beliefs beyond our conscious awareness.

The Spiritual Body

The most yang, ephemeral, and intangible aspect of the subtle body is the spiritual body. It is also referred to as the causal plane or the plane of destiny. The spiritual body is accessed through the delta state, which requires deep sleep or ritual. This is the aspect of our soul that existed before we came into physical form, and it is where all our life lessons are designed. It is the master blueprint of our lives. Some believe that we can access this blueprint through the Akashic records. Others believe that as humans, we can never truly know our full destiny. Healing the spiritual body comes from our own work connecting to the Divine, be it through prayer, divination, meditation, chanting, or ritual. Plant medicine at the level of the spiritual body includes offering a plant on an altar or shrine, or taking spiritual baths.

★★★

Yin and yang dance together and constantly seek balance in the universe. As you can see from the chart that follows, we use a yang state of awareness (beta) to access the most yin aspect of our being (the physical body); we can

---

11. *Odu Ifa* is the name for the divination system used in Ifa, which contains 256 energetic patterns. The priest will extract the proper verse of the story for the client to give archetypal insight into the question asked.

use the most yin state of awareness (delta) to access the most yang aspect of our being (the spiritual body).

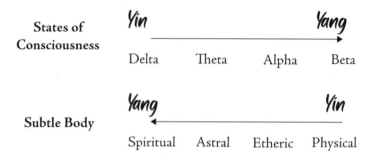

Hippocrates, known as the father of modern medicine, once said, "For this is the great error of our day, that the physicians separate the soul from the body."[12] This is a resounding endorsement for soul medicine! You will find that resources offered in this book focus primarily on the etheric and astral planes. They invite us to become efficient in accessing our alpha and theta states of consciousness as we work in the spaces between body and spirit. Soul medicine practices are universally available to us, no matter the condition of our physical body or what religion we follow.

Here is where I offer my disclaimer: the East Asian, Indigenous, and Diasporic healing systems on which this work is based are deep and vast. The assessment tools and soul medicine practices I offer are not intended to replace your doctor, your therapist, your intuition, or your spiritual/religious understandings. My hope is that as you develop your own relationship with the elements, you will be able to see, value, appreciate, and understand these potent forces of energy in our modern world. It is also my prayer that if you are reading this book, you will discover the soul medicine that resonates with you and supports your path to physical, emotional, mental, and spiritual healing.

---

12. Keith J. Karren, N. Lee Smith, and Kathryn J Gordon, *Mind/Body Health: The Effects of Attitudes, Emotions, and Relationships* (Boston: Pearson, 2014), 1.

Chapter 2
Working with the Elements

The self-assessment discovery prompts that follow will help you narrow down where to start your journey. Inspired by my teenage years taking personality quizzes in *Cosmo* magazine, this chapter will give you a peek into your inner world and which of the elements are at work in your life.

Now, let's use a four-step process to figure out which elements are most relevant for you, right now.

- Step One: Exploration *What are you ready to change?*
- Step Two: Emotions: *How do you know what needs your attention?*
- Step Three: Signatures: *What additional influence does an element have in your life?*
- Step Four: Purpose: *What is your why?*

Step One: Exploration

Let's start by figuring out *how* your qi is flowing. Where are you feeling in your element? Where do you need some support? Don't overthink your answer—just take a minute to rate a few key areas of your life according to the following scale:

0 = Not applicable.

1 = Yikes! This is a major source of stress.

2 = Hmm … I could use some support in this area.

3 = I have a handle on this, or know what changes I need to make.

4 = Good–This is really working for me.

5= Excellent–This aspect of my life is a source of joy and satisfaction!

Work/Career/School	
Living Situation	
Family Life	
Personal Romantic Relationships	
Diet/Exercise Regimen	
Creative Pursuits	
Physical Health	
Social Activism/Engagement	
Spirituality	
Finances	
Hobbies/Personal Interests	
Sex Life/Sexuality	
Parenting	
Social Life/Friendships	

As you take a look at your scores, you may already know what is calling for your attention. The areas that you scored a 4 or 5 are the areas where your Qi is most likely flowing, and you are probably feeling In Your Element! I hope you are taking time out to enjoy, celebrate, and send a prayer of gratitude up for those areas that are really working for you. But let's talk about those 1s, 2s, and 3s. Qi flowing? Not so much. You might even be surprised as you notice what's working—and what's not.

Let's take this assessment a step further. While looking at the numbers might give you some idea of what you're trying to change, your real life is not so … rational. Sometimes you *know* through and through that something needs to change, but you have *no desire* to work on it. And sometimes, something that on the surface feels like it's not a big deal can consume your energy and attention. Your heart has a mind of its own, so you might as well learn to listen to it. In your journal, take a moment to reflect on the following questions:

Step 1A: Reflection Questions: What are You Ready to Change?

- Based on the answers above, what is the one area of your life that is most calling for attention?
- What feels time-sensitive or urgent?
- What has your attention when you are trying to do other things?
- What are you inspired by, and/or has momentum?

Now comes the fun part. You are going to pick *one thing* to focus on for this cycle of inner soul work. How long is a cycle? That's up to you! It can be a week, a month, a season—whatever feels like the right amount of time to dedicate consistent, loving attention. Traditionally speaking, emotional soul shifts happen in cycles of twenty-eight to thirty days, so that is the recommended time frame for the tools described in the chapters that follow. But you are the expert in your life, so you know best what timing will work for you.

Also, don't stress yourself out about picking the "right" thing. I subscribe to the Mosaic philosophy of healing. Yes, I made that up, but it works. Think about a mosaic. When you stand back you see one big picture, but when you look closely, you see that there's actually a million tiny photos that create the full image. Our life is a mosaic, and you are the big picture made up of tiny images of your experience. This means you can take any one of those tiny images—your relationship, your spirituality, your parenting, or your career—and you will still be working on you. As you change one small image, the larger image of yourself and how you show up in the world will also change. That's how soul work happens—one beautiful snapshot at a time.

Step 1B: Set Your Intention

- For the next _____ (days, weeks, or months) you commit to transforming _____.
- Why are you ready to transform this area of your life?

In your journal, write down a clear statement of intention for this phase of your soul work.

Step Two: Emotions

My favorite author is Octavia Butler (she is one of the few authors I do read cover to cover). In her freakily realistic sci-fi book *Parable of the Sower*, the lead character creates a religion called Earthseed based on the following scripture:

"Everything you touch, you change.

Everything you change, changes you.

The only lasting truth is change."[13]

Nothing could be more true, as far as qi is concerned. The nature of qi is to move, to transform, to wax and wane. As you look at how you rated your life above, you know I'm not lying. That area you rated a 5 today could have been a 1 a year ago. That 3 might have been a 5 before yesterday's argument with your love. Which means that area rated a 1—no matter how stressful and stuck it feels right now—also has the potential to change. Our lives are dynamic, not static. We fluctuate between being happy and sad, accepting and outraged, inspired and disillusioned. Every day is different, and every day *we* are different.

How do we know when and where our life qi is blocked? It's easy. Our emotions clue us in with feelings of frustration, confusion, sadness, anxiety, anger, grief, and all the feels. The five elements teach us how to use our emotions as a guide, directing us to the areas in our lives where our qi needs more flow. The next step in your exploration is tuning in to your feelings, which you can think of as the changing climate in your emotional landscape. We all experience many emotions, and they can change from moment to moment. But often when we are ready to make a change in our lives, there are one or two core emotions that take center stage. They can sometimes be the default emotion that gets stirred, regardless of the actual situation. Those emotions may even seep into other aspects of our lives. We can tune in to and learn from those emotions that are persistent, stuck, unprocessed, or creating challenges in our lives. We can also pay attention to an emotion whose intensity surprises us, catches us off guard, or gets expressed out of proportion to the actual situation.

Take a moment, and take a deep breath. Now, call into mind your goal for this cycle of soul work. When you draw your attention inward and focus on this area of your life *as it is now*, how does it feel?

---

13. Octavia E. Butler, *Parable of the Sower* (New York: Grand Central Publishing, 2019), 3.

Step 2 Reflection Questions: How Do I Feel?

+ Are there any emotions that come up more frequently than others?
+ Are there any emotions you try to suppress or deny?
+ How have you been expressing these emotions?
+ Which element most closely aligns with how you feel?

Water	Wood	Fire	Earth	Metal
Fear	Anger	Love or Loveless	Worry	Sadness
Anxiety	Rage	Vulnerable	Overthinking	Grief
Panic	Irritability/ Agitation	Joyful/ Joyless	Empathy	Disappointed
Paralyzed	Depression	Betrayal	Ungrounded	Shame
Timid/Shy	Hopelessness	Disconnected	Unsupported	Nostalgic
Nervous	Oppressed	Heartbroken	Procrastinating	Heavy
Hesitant	Stuck	Distrust/ Suspicion	Indecisive	Unworthy
Confused	Frustrated	Mania/ Insomnia	Frazzled	Deflated
Antisocial	Impatient	Isolated	Disorganized	Devastated
	Mood Swings	Shock	Overwhelmed	Disillusioned

Each element governs a specific movement of qi, as well as certain emotional climates. In this system, our emotions are not bad, even if they are uncomfortable. We may prefer sunny weather, but the rain is important. We can stand in the rain (cue New Edition[14]) when we have the right tools—umbrella, boots, flip-flops, or a bathing suit depending on your cultural upbringing. The same is true with our emotions—we can make better space for them when we understand that they are our allies pointing to where we

---

14. "Can You Stand the Rain" is one of R&B group New Edition's most popular songs, peaking on Urban BillBoard in the 1990s. Say the words "stand" and "rain" in close proximity to any Black forty-plus-year-old and they will break into song, at least in their head.

need support. The goal is not to numb our emotions or even to make us "feel better." Instead, we can observe—with curiosity and compassion—the movement of our emotions as they flow through us. As Pastor Greg from Celebration Spiritual Center eloquently posted on Instagram, "You are the sky. Not the weather."[15]

Step Three: Signatures

Each of the elements is an archetype, meaning that each relates to universal themes that transcend time, place, and culture. You can also think of these elements as spheres of influence. Each element governs (by association) certain areas of life that it controls or influences. In Western medicine is a direct, linear relationship between a cause (such as a bacteria or virus) and the effect (a cold or flu). But Indigenous and Diasporic medicine follows a different kind of logic. Rather than linear time, our inner soul work relies on synchronicity, coincidence, symbols, associations, and patterns. Instead of looking for reasons, we look for signatures. These signatures put the stamp of an element on our life, creating currents of connection between things that seem unrelated.

For example, consider my patient with Liver Qi stagnation (a popular diagnosis here in New York City due to the intensity and pace of the environment). Here are some signatures of the Wood element that are showing up in her life:

- Feeling stuck and frustrated at work, as well as feeling powerless in the face of constant microaggressions
- Working long hours
- Smoking weed to decompress and to release her tension
- Not having time to exercise
- Having lots of arguments with her husband, who doesn't understand why she is always so tense
- Feeling less time, inspiration, and desire to work on the creative projects in her heart

---

15. Greg Stamper (@iamgregstamper), Instagram June 16, 2020. https://www.instagram.com/iamgregstamper/.

In this example, her experiences are tied together through the archetype of the Wood element. Encoded in that tapestry are also the gifts and blessings of the Wood element. These circumstances align as an incentive for my patient to tap into her creative genius, her authentic communication, and her ability to set clear and effective boundaries, which are also signatures of the Wood element.

On the grid that follows, place a check next to the elemental signatures that relate to your mission statement and arena of inner work this cycle:

Water

_____ Resources (having enough time, money or emotional support)

_____ Ancestry/Family Roots

_____ Intuition

_____ Willpower

_____ Home

_____ Safety and Security

Wood

_____ Work/Career/Entrepreneurship

_____ Leadership

_____ Social Justice/Activism

_____ Conflict

_____ Boundaries

_____ Public Speaking or Creative Expression

Fire

_____ Relationships

_____ Partnerships

_____ Intimacy

_____ Sex & Sensuality

_____ Friendships/Social Life

_____ Visibility/Networking

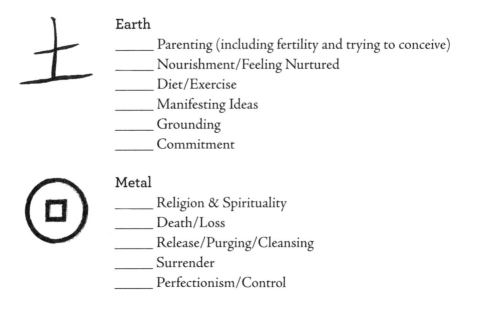

Earth
_____ Parenting (including fertility and trying to conceive)
_____ Nourishment/Feeling Nurtured
_____ Diet/Exercise
_____ Manifesting Ideas
_____ Grounding
_____ Commitment

Metal
_____ Religion & Spirituality
_____ Death/Loss
_____ Release/Purging/Cleansing
_____ Surrender
_____ Perfectionism/Control

Step 3 Reflection Questions: What Influence Does an Element Have in Your Life?

+ Which element most relates thematically to your inner work?
+ Which signatures of this element are reflected in your experience?

Step Four: Purpose

Life happens, and try as we might, we can't always know the rhyme or reason. We've experienced unexpected blessings that we don't believe we've earned. We've come face-to-face with heartache we tried to avoid. We've experienced grief that has tested the limits of our faith. We've experienced love that explodes in ecstasy.

A few years ago, I joined a weight management program in which I was asked to identify my *why* for joining. Well, duh…to lose weight! But then they asked me why again—and again and again—until I got down to a core value that could motivate me each morning. I wanted to feel vibrant, connected, and alive. This was an important step for me, because the lifestyle changes I needed to make were *hard*. And shedding some pounds by itself just simply wasn't enough motivation. I felt beautiful in my body, so losing pounds for external appearance didn't mean enough to me. My *why* had to be tied to a deeper meaning, value, and purpose. Experiencing myself as a more sensual, vibrant, and orgasmic being? Yes, YES, and YASSSSSSSSS! That *why* kept me focused when I was discouraged after slipups and resentful of the process, and even when I actually forgot why I had started the whole damn thing in the first place. And that *why* also led me into a deep exploration of the Fire element. As you'll learn in chapter 5, the Fire element helps us discover our sensuality, passion, and joy.

The gifts of the elements become our "why," but they are not the cause of ill or good fortune. Instead, they offer a glimpse of our potential for greatness, our next level for being more fully and authentically ourselves. They help us imagine who we would be if we were living fully in our element. The gifts and blessings listed on the chart below are just a small sampling of the beautiful becoming that is in store for us when we harmonize an element within us.

Water	Wood	Fire	Earth	Metal
Rest	Authenticity	Love	Health	Inspiration
Rejuvenation	Confidence	Connection	Support	Spirit
Intuition	Agency	Intimacy	Gratitude	Serenity
Introspection	Self-Actualization	Joy	Family	Reverence
Inner Calm	Righteousness	Sensuality	Community	Mindfulness
Wisdom	Self-Expression	Vitality	Understanding	Transcendence
Insight	Courage	Compassion	Empathy	Worthiness

Step 4 Reflection: What Is Your "Why"?

Use the chart above to help you answer the following questions:
- Why do you want to transform this area of your life?
- What possibilities are you welcoming?
- If a genie could offer you the gifts of one of these elements, which would you choose and why?

★★★

You just did a lot of work! Take a moment, take a breath, take a nap, or take a day or two to sit with what you just discovered. When you're ready, come on back. Next, we'll get to know the soul lessons of each of the elements, which will help you make big changes—inside and out.

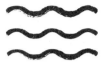

Chapter 3
Sacred Waters

Water is the master shapeshifter because it has so many forms. There are still waters that run deep. There are crashing waves on the shore that ebb and flow. Water is the tsunami, the gentle stream, fresh water, salt water, and womb water. No matter its form, water equals life.

Water Element Signatures

We experience the archetypal qualities of the Water element through the following signatures:

- Season: Winter
- Phase: Seed
- Color: Blue/black
- Energetic: Sinks qi
- Core Emotion: Fear
- Sound: Groaning
- Meridians: Kidney and Bladder

Season: Winter

When I gaze through my window on a cold winter day, I see trees standing naked and still beneath the weight of the snow. My rose bush looks like a big bundle of dead branches. But the truth is there's a lot going on beneath the surface. Rather than being focused on blossoming her beautiful roses, she has channeled all of her resources inward. All trees do this in the winter. Instead of sending their energy out to their leaves, the trees wisely sink their nourishing capacity into their core and into their roots.

Animals also pull their resources inward to hibernate in the deep sleep of winter. You won't find a cat, a rat (this is New York, people!), raccoon, or any other animal once the temperatures start to plunge. And like our furry friends, during winter—the season of the Water element—we find ourselves sleeping more, valuing quiet and stillness, reflecting on the year's lessons and blessings. Cuddling under thick blankets becomes more inviting than a night out. In the silence and stillness, we can hear the whispers of our inner wisdom. In the Water element, we access our intuition and learn to value the messages that emerge from deep within.

Phase: Seed

In the cycle of organic life, the Water element is represented by the seed— deep, dark, planted, and hidden in the mysterious womb of the earth. Within the seed there is the entire blueprint of what it is to become. It is full of potential—within the acorn, there is already the mighty oak. It has its destiny encoded into every cell, and the life journey of the acorn is the process of becoming an oak.

Like the acorn, we are also born as seeds of potential. The Water element helps us to tap into that master blueprint for our lives. We gain insight into that encoded blueprint by tapping into everything that has come before us— our ancestors, our family tree, our lineage, our past, and the collective consciousness of humanity. Deep study of philosophical ideas or history, metaphysical wisdom, and the mystery sciences are also in the realm of the Water element.

Of the five phases, the Water element represents the beginning *before* the beginning. It represents a phase of incubation, like the womb waters before birth. We tap into Water when we have an idea that is still forming but we are not yet ready to share or act on it. This is the Water element's *potent, pregnant pause.* Acting prematurely would weaken its potency; not sharing at the right time results in stagnation or missed opportunity. Water is also present when we feel something in our emotional depths but do not yet have the language to express it. Like a seed, the Water element teaches us to honor the deep mystery of being secret, unrevealed, and belonging to darkness.

Color: Blue/Black

Though we often illustrate water with shades of blue, Water in Five Element theory is classically associated with a dark blue-black color. This black is like the mysterious color between rocks or the entrance to a cave, the sheen of wet pavement, and the night sky of a new moon. I never quite understood the color of Water until the winter night I took the Haverstraw–Ossining Ferry over the Hudson River. There, I experienced the Water element as I imagined the ancients once did—without the interference of electricity. In the cold, dark, and quiet night, the river waves rolled like black silk. Black draws itself within, evoking the introspective, mysterious feeling of the Water element.

Energetic: Sinks Qi

The energetic direction of water is downward and inward, as water always seeks the deepest level. Imagine if you were to knock over a glass of water. The water would first roll off the table and onto the floor. If there is a hole in the floor, the water will seep into the hole and keep falling, down, down, down. We could imagine that if there were no obstruction and enough water, it would keep descending all the way to the center of Earth. The Water element surrenders to the force of gravity, rooting us to the earth and holding us safely here.

Core Emotion: Fear

The emotion associated with the Water element is fear, which also draws qi downward. A great example of how fear sinks qi is when a child is scared and pees on themselves. It's that sinking feeling we get when we know, instinctively, that something is about to take a turn for the worse. In Water's depths, we are confronted with our needs for safety, security, and survival. The Water element gifts us with the ability to assess risk, cultivate cautious awareness of our surroundings, and bring focused attention to the present moment. In its healthiest expression, fear gifts us with the capacity for caution, instinctual action, and intuition.

What does healthy fear look like? Fear is that instinctual response that allows us to jump out of the way of a car speeding toward us before we have time to think about it. Healthy fear calls to mind the image of a mama bird with her babies in a nest nearby. Mama is watching, waiting, cautious, alert, and ready to respond. This is an appropriate stance when we find ourselves in an emotionally or physically threatening situation. That awareness and readiness is part of the natural stress response meant to keep us alive! But outside of a threatening situation, hypervigilance and alertness quickly escalate into anxiety, suspicion, or panic. The fear can also manifest as mistrust of people or opportunities.

Without appropriate fear, we can be reckless, either from a sense of invincibility or an apathetic attitude toward life. Complete lack of fear—best described as reckless abandon—is a manifestation of Water out of balance. When we are uprooted and completely disconnected from Water's gravity, we might find ourselves spinning dangerously out of control. Water brings us the overwhelming feeling that we might lose it at any moment. The Water element restores a deep sense of trust that assures us that we can, in fact, stay the course. Others seek out Water's adrenaline rush through skydiving, bungee jumping, overworking to the brink of exhaustion, or dangerous relationships. The Water element brings awareness of our desperate and destructive impulses, and can be a catalyst to seeking out the support we truly need.

The Water element also gifts us with wisdom. My daughter is a great example. When she was a toddler, she absolutely refused to sit down in the bathtub. She would lock her knees, and there was nothing that I or her 6'2", 190 pound father could do to assure her that the water was safe. She would tolerate us washing her with a sponge and rinsing her with water in a cup, but sitting down in the bathtub was not an option. She engaged her Water meridians by rooting through her feet, locking her knees, and holding her ground. This habit continued until we went to a pool party for one of her cousins. I watched as she carefully observed (like a bird watching over her nest) the other children as they splashed and played in the pool. Following their lead, she gradually walked far enough into the water for it to cover her knees, then her belly button, and then finally she was sitting in the water having a great time (at which point I became the watchful bird)! We never had a problem getting her to sit down in the bathtub again. The wisdom of her experience helped her overcome her fear.

Fear can take many forms but often wears a disguise. Like anger, it is an emotion that we may not admit having to ourselves or others. We might lock our knees and present a tough exterior to hide our fear. We might give reasons to justify our actions, not even realizing that fear lies at the root. Listed below are a few variations of fear:

Fear	Shyness	Doubt
Terror	Anxiety	Insecurity
Paralysis	Apprehension	Suspicion
Timidity	Trepidation	Panic
Depression	Uncertainty	

Sound: Groaning

The sound of the Water element in a person's voice has a groaning quality. An example of this groan or croak is when your first words in the morning are "that was a good sleep," before fully waking up. The sound of Water has a characteristic sinking quality, either in its low tones or in a voice that falls and sinks at the ends of sentences. Musically, we can evoke the feeling of Water with songs that carry the vibration of sinking to the depths, slow rhythms that evoke stillness or trance, deep bass, and notes that accumulate in the lower register. There is sometimes a sense of foreboding and warning in Water's music, like the eerie soundtrack in a horror movie. My students keep me young, and often will reference the haunting vibes of trap music.

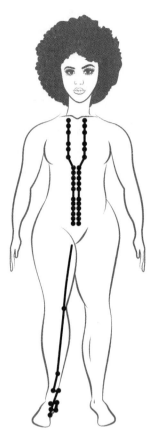

3.1 Kidney Meridian

Meridians: Kidney and Bladder

The Kidneys and the Bladder are the organs associated with the Water element, along with the womb and the adrenals. The Kidney meridian [**Figure 3.1**] starts at the sole of the foot, encircles the inner ankle, rises through the inner thigh, penetrates the womb, and ascends to the chest. The Bladder meridian starts in the corner of the inner eye, travels along the top of the head, [**Figure 3.2**] descends along the back, buttocks, and hamstring, around the outer ankle, and ends at the tip of the pinky toe [**Figure 3.3**]. When the Water element meridians are compromised, some of the physical symptoms we experience include:

+ Back pain (especially in the lower back)
+ Fatigue and exhaustion
+ Headaches
+ Difficulty inhaling with deep breaths
+ Dryness (skin, mouth, vaginal, etc.)
+ Urinary incontinence
+ Fertility challenges
+ Low libido
+ Cavities and teeth problems

In yoga, poses that stretch the hamstrings and align the spine help to nurture the meridians of Water element. We can practice the Water element's rooting down energetic with standing or balancing postures, when we imagine our roots sinking down out of the standing foot and rooting us into the earth. We also access the Water element in postures that invite introspection, and evoke a sense of safety and protection. Keeping our feet covered with socks, using heating pads on our lower abdomen or low back, and taking salt baths are all ways to nourish the Water meridians.

Soul Lesson 1: Create an Oasis

Each person deserves a day away in which no problems are confronted, no solutions are searched for. Each of us needs to withdraw from the cares which will not withdraw from us.
—*Maya Angelou*

The ancients knew that there are two kinds of will—my will, and thy will. My will, or my personal will, is based on my desires, intentions, and personal goals. Then there is the cosmic will, in which my personal aspiration is but a single thread in the tapestry of the universe. When we align our personal will to cosmic will, we experience ease in the manifestation of our desires. Our actions are equally met by the universe's desire to meet our needs. When the two are not aligned, we experience limitations, obstructions, and delays. It feels like a fight to swim upstream against the current. Water teaches us how to find an oasis in the upstream battle. The oasis is a safe place for us to rest, reassess, and realign.

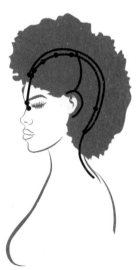

3.2 Bladder Meridian Points on Head

When our personal will is healthy, we set goals and take action. Our determination and drive align to lead us to success. I admire these folks whose seeing, saying, and doing all happen in one swoop. But, when our personal will is overactive, we plow through our life driven by an unbalanced desire to accomplish. Our will to succeed leads to working extremely long hours at the sacrifice of relationships, our body's needs for food or rest, and our spiritual life. Our overactive will might also make us unreceptive and unable to see anything that doesn't fit with our plan. We try to use physical force, personal power, manipulation, external resources, or sheer will to make things happen, with little trust that our needs will be met without us doing the absolute most.

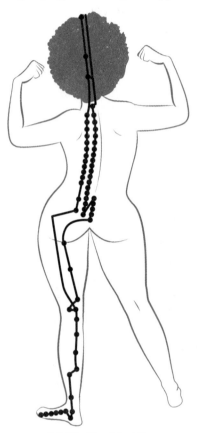

3.3 Bladder Meridian

On the other end of the spectrum, our personal will can tank and we have very little motivation. The painting *Blue Monday* by Annie Lee perfectly illustrates this feeling. In the painting, a woman sits on the edge of her bed, shoulders heavily slumped, as if standing would require more energy than she can possibly muster. Let's just say the "get up and go" got up and went! In this state, we feel like we don't have the energy or time to handle all the responsibilities on our plate. Projects (and people) that once excited us feel exhausting. We procrastinate as we let our goals collect dust on our mental shelf.

In Five Element theory, *zhi* is a concept that does not quite translate into English. It is sometimes defined as the will, personal will, or motive force. I describe zhi as the bridge between the personal will and cosmic will, between my will and thy will. And to cross that bridge, we have to call on the Water element. Through the Water element, we gain the wisdom that teaches us what resources to use and what to save, when to act and when to wait. We learn the simple elegance of being in alignment with our destiny so that we don't have to rely exclusively on our willpower to get what we need. We can trust that what we need and desire is flowing toward us, so that we can balance effort and ease.

Reflection Questions

How well are you creating an oasis? Take a moment to reflect on the following questions in your journal:

+ In what areas of your life are you pushing yourself beyond your limits? Why?
+ When are you aware you're running on "E"?
+ How do you refill your tank when you're depleted?
+ How hard is it for you to press PAUSE or even STOP?
+ What spiritual lessons need time, patience, or perseverance to integrate?

Flower Essences for Creating an Oasis

Flower essences that support our ability to create a soul oasis include:

+ Oak for honoring our limitations
+ Aloe Vera for recovering from burnout
+ Olive for replenishing reserves
+ Sweet Chestnut for sweet surrender

Oak: Honor Limitations—Oak flower essence teaches us how to recognize our limitations. Remember when we discussed the acorn having everything it needs encoded within to achieve its destiny? We are the same. We are born with the blueprint and the innate power to achieve our destiny, not one thing more, not one thing less. The problem is we can deplete the resources we have doing the wrong things. I personally have a superwoman complex that kicks in and makes me want to take on any- and everything—creative projects, men I want to date who are also projects.... Sigh. But then I have to ask myself: Do I really have the time or energy to take this on? Even more importantly, *am I supposed to take this on?* Oak helps us take inventory of our inner and outer resources, and reassess our limitations so that we can be clear on how to use what we got to get what we want.

I know my patients would benefit from Oak flower essence when they say things like, "If I don't do it, no one will," or, "If I don't take care of this, everything will fall apart." They end up running on an empty tank. And it may actually be true that things will get super messy if they take a step back. To which the Water element says in a grand, definitive voice, "So be it." Oak teaches us how to yield to our limitations and let go of the struggle. Oak allows us to honor the limitations of our destiny not as a negative curse but as a positive blessing. With Oak, we learn how to reallocate our inner resources—our intention, attention, gifts, and effort—to those things which are truly meant to be.

Aloe Vera: Balance the Burnout—The aloe vera plant is a beautiful example of balancing Fire and Water. Within the leaves of the aloe plant is a soft, gooey, succulent gel that nourishes and soothes. Most of us don't get to see aloe's flower blossoms, which are bright yellow, spiky, vibrant, and quite fiery. As a flower essence, Aloe Vera helps to balance our brilliant, creative nature with the need to replenish. It's an essence we call on when we have been producing so much that we are either tanked out or about to tank out.

There are moments when our passion and creativity consume us. We may stay up all night working on projects or even lie in bed unable to sleep because of the ideas and inspiration flooding our minds. We may skip meals, skimp on sleep, or lose track of time as we deeply immerse ourselves in our work or creative flow. Sometimes we recognize when burning the candle at both ends is a problem and feel the weight of overwhelm. Other times, the rush of adrenaline and creativity feel incredible. The energy and drive can sustain us for a while, but inevitably there comes a point when everything will crash. In those moments of burnout, we feel disconnected and unable to access our creative spark.

Aloe Vera flower essence can support us on either side of this polarity. If we recognize (or someone gently points out) that we are in overdrive, aloe vera encourages us to find balance in our schedule. It replenishes the heart so that we can awaken its sensitivity to our soul and body's needs without disrupting our creative flow. Aloe Vera coaxes us to find joy and sweetness in the creative process, instead of overemphasizing the outcome. If we are already burned out and lacking inspiration, Aloe Vera gently sparks the heart to reconnect with our creativity. Its role is to encourage us to reorganize our lives so that we can anchor our creative inspiration without becoming depleted.

Olive: Replenish Reserves—We call on Olive flower essence when we are capital T Tired. This is not the "I need a nap" kind of tired—this is the kind of exhaustion we feel when no amount of sleep would do us any good. It's a fatigue that we feel deep in our bones, when even the smallest tasks seem impossible. In addition to feeling physically tired, we may have a low mood or a hard time managing stress. Imagine driving a car that is running out of gas, but the next gas station is still twenty miles down the road. You keep driving, the gas light comes on, and you know you are out of gas. But there's still five miles to go. You get to the gas station…and it's *closed*. The next one is two miles away. Agh! If the car could talk, it would look at you and say, "Are you CRAZY right now!? I've got nothing left!" At this point, you are running on fumes and determination. That's the kind of fatigue I'm talking about that calls for Olive flower essence.

I use Olive to support many of the clients I see in my practice, especially my postpartum mamas, my entrepreneurial bosses taking care of their parents, and my single sisters working full-time jobs while simultaneously home-schooling because of COVID. When I ask them if they can take a day off or go on a vacation, they look at me like I am crazy. "How?! When?!" they ask. It's a question I can't answer, because everything I suggest sounds impossible. There is too much to do and no one else can do it. Right? But then Olive flower essence works her magic and says, "We are out of gas and need to fuel up—let me teach you how." When working with Olive, we can expect insight into how to integrate rest and replenishment into our routine.

Sometimes, it helps us to see (for the first time) how exhausted we truly are and the lifestyle changes we need to make because of it. This is the difference between flower essences and other forms of plant medicine. When feeling exhausted, we might turn to herbs that help us build energy, such as ginseng or sea moss. We might integrate energy-building foods or supplements. Herbal remedies, fortifying foods, and essential oils can help refill the gas in the tank. But Olive flower essence is going to offer insight into *when* and *where* in our lives to refuel, as well as how not to burn that fuel so quickly. That could mean a vacation or integrating more downtime in the workweek.

Maybe it's a salt bath or glass of wine (or both!) at the end of the day. It could mean rearranging our schedule to get more sleep, or taking a break from social media. Perhaps it's recognizing that certain people drain our energy and we are called to renegotiate the ways in which we interact. The beauty of working with flower essences is that there is no one size that fits all—the insights awaken from within and are applied within the context of our own lives. As a flower essence, Olive helps us honor our need to replenish, and helps us discover the best way to make that happen.

Sweet Chestnut: Sweet surrender—In a tech-driven yang society, we want what we want when we want it. We celebrate new insights, aha moments, and epiphanies as we grow in spiritual awareness. It takes a slow and unpredictable process to embody that awareness into experience, and that can be painful. The "dark night of the soul" refers to those moments when we are invited to integrate spiritual truths into our lives. This integration requires being in the darkness and feeling the labor pains of birthing a new way of being in the world. This feels like heartbreak. Sometimes it feels like drowning.

In archetypal depth psychology, this process is called the *Connunctio* and the *Nigredo*.[16] The Connunctio is yang in nature. It represents new awareness, enlightenment, and epiphany. During the Connunctio, our consciousness expands. But as nature's law would have it, every Conunctio is followed by the Nigredo, which essentially knocks us back on our ass. In the Nigredo, we are forced to ask: "What needs to change in my life for this insight to manifest?" The reorganization takes time, is slow, and requires surrender, stillness, patience, introspection.

Here's the Connunctio and Nigredo in a real-life example: Last year I participated in an Isefa, a rite of passage in the Ifa tradition. I was almost levitating after three days of wearing white, meditating, praying, and receiving insight into my destiny. I was empowered and ready to take over the world, or at least my corner of it. My heart felt expanded and open, like any- and everything was possible: love, marriage, wealth, prosperity, health, and even

---

16. Lorie Eve Dechar and Benjamin Fox, *The Alchemy of Inner Work: A Guide for Turning Illness and Suffering into True Health and Well-Being* (Newburyport, MA: Weiser Books, 2021), 16–27.

this book. We're talking Connunctio on a thousand—I can't remember a time I felt so clear and inspired.

Do you know what happened the following week? I learned that the man I had been seeing for almost two years was cheating on me. When I approached him about the woman who was posting embarrassing comments under our social media photos, he responded with a coldness that made him almost unrecognizable to me. I was devastated; it felt like the rug was pulled out from under me. Can I tell you I went to a dark place? *Man,* it was *dark* in there! As the relationship exploded, I questioned everything about my worthiness and my capacity for love. But the darkness didn't stop there—it spread to include other areas of my life, too. I questioned my capacity to be a good mother, if I had anything worthwhile to say in a book, the trajectory of my entire career, and my purpose in life. Anything and everything that felt great two weeks before suddenly felt clouded and obscure. The clarity from Isefa was replaced with confusion and self-doubt, and my newly opened heart closed as I isolated myself to tend to my wounds. My entire life needed a reset if I was going to actualize any of the brilliance promised. That, my friends, is the Nigredo.

Sweet Chestnut is the flower essence that supports us through these dark moments of inner turmoil. Consider the caterpillar, which we know goes through a beautiful transformational process to become a butterfly. But what does it feel like inside of the cocoon? Like death, I'm sure, as everything it knows dissolves into nothingness. In that darkness, the only light is its own heart, a beat that grows stronger and more luminescent as it shapes into a new form. Soon it will beat its wings to break free, but not a moment before its time. If it escapes the contractive pressure of the cocoon too soon, its wings will not be strong enough to survive in the world. Without this necessary pain, it will not become who it is meant to be.

In the Water element, we feel that discomfort and darkness of transformation. It's that moment when we've unearthed the wound, the trauma, or the painful parts of ourselves that need healing, but cannot yet know the medicine or solution. We might turn to drugs, alcohol, food, lovers, or denial to cope with or escape the pain of the uncomfortable reshaping. Like labor pains or contractions, they are reminders that something is about to be born, but it's not the time *just* yet—and that timing cannot be rushed.

It's freaking scary in there. We have to trust. We have to surrender. We have to endure the pressure. We are invited to lean into the wisdom that there is nothing we will be given that we can't handle. Sweet Chestnut flower essence supports us as we reconnect to strength we did not know we had, wisdom we did not know existed, and courage we did not think was possible. It helps us to call on deep wells of perseverance and patience as we swim in the waters of the unknown, especially when we believe we are at the limits of our inner capacity to cope. Sweet Chestnut also restores our faith and connection to our spiritual guidance, no matter our religious orientation. It transforms our angst into deep trust that all is well, even when we don't have all the answers.

Embodied Practice: Viparita Karani (Waterfall Pose)

Affirmation: I take time to replenish

Lie on your back and extend your legs toward the sky. For more support, rest your legs against the wall, and/or place a yoga block under your sacrum. Make sure your knees are slightly bent to your comfort level and not locked.

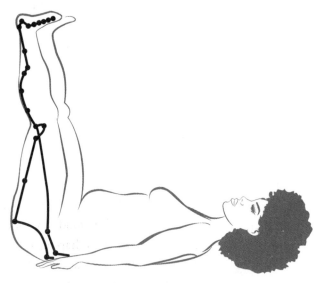

Pictured with the Bladder Meridian

Flex your toes. Envision a gentle waterfall flowing from your feet and pooling in a gentle lake in your lower abdomen. Imagine that this lake, in the center of your being, is a place where you can relax, unwind, and replenish.

Close your eyes and rest as you repeat the affirmation: *I take time to replenish.* If your schedule is overfull, give yourself permission to rest in this replenishing pose a few extra minutes. Notice any internal dialogue that resists this moment for yourself.

Soul Lesson 2: Connect to the Source

Do not be afraid to disappear—from it, from us, for a while…
and see what comes to you in the silence.
—Emmy Award winning writer Michaela Coel

The Water element helps us process the world through all of the states of awareness and perception that we have available beyond our normal, waking mind. How can we turn up the volume of the messages from our dreams, our intuition, our heart's knowing? How do we turn down the noise of other people's expectations and advice? Turning down the external noise means turning down the static—spending less time online or on social media, or less time socializing so that we can get quiet enough to hear.

Sometimes we get so intent on knowing what to do and when to do it that we miss a valuable moment that the Water element offers. And that is the invaluable moment when we admit to ourselves three magical words: *I don't know.* That moment of not knowing is a precious part of our humanity. Sure, we might hit up Google, call a friend, make countless spreadsheets, or go super metaphysical by turning to divination, prayer, or our astrology chart (all of which are governed by the Water element, by the way), but there is a sacred moment right before we do any of those things—the moment that we acknowledge that *we don't know.* That is the moment that allows us to surrender to our destiny, and to acknowledge that we are here for a purpose that is beyond what our logical, intellectual human minds can perceive. In moments of not knowing, we are reminded that the truth does not lie in just what we can see, but in the unseen forces that are guiding our steps. That is the sacred source.

We call on the Water element to help us redirect our gaze inward. In some cases, Water causes us to increase our spiritual practices—more prayer, more chanting, more meditation, more stillness, more silence. In some cases, the Water element will encourage us to clean up and clear the clutter and distractions in our lives. At other times, the Water element will inspire us to begin a journaling practice, start an artistic hobby, or go into nature or some other space where we can listen to our internal waters. Whatever path we choose, the Water element is there to guide us gently (or forcibly) back to ourselves.

Reflection Questions

Are you connected to your source? Take a moment to reflect on the following questions in your journal:

- How do you feel about being quiet, still, or alone?
- How much noise surrounds you? How much noise are you creating?
- Can you hear your inner knowing? Do you trust it?
- How and when do you surrender to not knowing? Are there areas of your life that are asking you to surrender now?
- What activities bring you serenity?
- What practices give you insight into "divine design"?
- How comfortable are you swimming in the waters of the unknown?
- What areas of your life are calling for you to trust other ways of perceiving and knowing?

Flower Essences for Connecting to the Source

The following flower essences support our ability to access knowing from beyond our logical and rational mind:

- Angelica for listening to ancestors and spirit guides
- Cerato for listening to intuition
- Mugwort for listening to dreams

Angelica: Listen to Your Spiritual Guides—Angelica is such a powerful essence, and it is so resonant with the Water element that it plays a prominent role in each of the Water element formulas. Patricia Kaminski, founder of the Flower Essence Society, shares the following affirmation for angelica:

"My angel guides me in life. My angel protects my holy purpose."[17] Whether we call on our ancestors, Jesus, guardian angels, the Divine Masters, Orisa, or all of the above, Angelica connects us to the light beings that are in charge of our guidance and protection.

In *Isese Spirituality Workbook: The Ancestral Wisdom of the Orisa Tradition*, Dr. Ayele Kumari describes the African concept of the *Ori*.[18] The Ori is the deity in charge of your consciousness, or head. Your Ori witnessed the destiny your spirit agreed to before coming to Earth. The tradition explains that when we get to Earth, we forget our destiny. We can connect to our Ori, also represented as the crown chakra, for guidance. The Ori gives us hints when we're going astray and when we're on the right path. When we're on the right path, doors seem to open as if by magic. There is synchronicity and an internal feeling of alignment. And when we're off our path, something doesn't feel quite right. We might feel it in the pit of our stomach, or as a gnawing sensation that things aren't going the way they should. In more extreme cases, we find ourselves at dead ends where we bump our heads against the wall.

Angelica attunes us to the subtle nudges, whispers, and urgings of our ancestors and our spiritual guides. It is a flower essence that helps us open the channels of receptivity so that we can hear messages more clearly. We feel angelica's magic whenever something unexpected shows up that was exactly what we were looking for. We feel her magic when we sense a gentle reminder that something or someone is looking out for us. Angelica helps us to feel the safety and protection from the spiritual realm. Sometimes we may get a clear image or insight into who or what is supporting us, and other times Angelica awakens a vague feeling or memory, a subtle heart lift, or the comforting awareness that we are not alone.

Soul Medicine Practice: Receptive Channel

To support your work with Angelica flower essence, I recommend the following exercise to become a "Receptive Channel":

---

17. *Affirm a Flower Affirmation Deck*, "Angelica" card. Flower Essence Society (FES), www.fesflowers.com.

18. Ayele Kumari, *The Isese Spirituality Workbook: The Ancestral Wisdom of the Orisa Tradition* (Self-published, 2020).

Step 1: Observe

Observe what is happening in your life. Take note of what feels blocked or limited and what feels open and expansive.

Step 2: Ask

Create a question for which you are seeking guidance, wisdom, or advice. Send it out through prayer, ritual, altar work, or meditation.

Step 3: Receive and Record

The answer to your question/s may come through dreams, synchronicities, breakthroughs, epiphanies, revelations, and serendipitous events. Pay attention to songs that you can't get out of your head, unexpected advice, and anything out of the ordinary that catches your attention. Have a sacred place to record these answers in the many ways they may show up. Even if something doesn't seem like a direct response to your question, record anything that you intuitively feel may be relevant or offering insight into your inner world.

Step 4: Confirm

Do the answers that you are receiving feel true? Do they resonate? Check in for an inner sense of alignment, or use tools from your personal spiritual practice for confirmation.

Step 5: Act

Acknowledge that you've received and accepted the message by sharing it with a friend, journaling, creating art and symbols, ritual, and/or an action or commitment.

Cerato: Listen to Your Intuition—Can you remember a time that you felt strongly called to do something but couldn't find a rhyme or reason for the impulse? What did you do in that moment? Did you trust yourself or did you talk yourself out of what you were feeling? Or, have you ever had an experience when, looking back, you wished you had trusted your gut? Cerato is the flower essence that helps us not only listen to our inner voice and intuition but also trust and act on what we hear—even if it goes against what our logic and reason are telling us.

I was definitely in a Cerato situation when a little inner voice suggested that I go to acupuncture school. At the time, I was confused about the next steps in my path, and asking the universe for a sign. That confusion can be pretty typical of those who need a little Cerato flower essence in their life. I learned that acupuncture programs cost upward of $70,000, and that it would take almost three years to complete the master of science degree. At that point, I decided that there was *no way* I was going to acupuncture school! My daughter was still in diapers, and my immediate family lived more than three hours away. I had a full-time job. I didn't have the time or the money. And yet…I knew deep down inside that despite the odds, somehow acupuncture school was right for me.

Trusting that inner voice and that intuitive push turned out to be one of my best decisions. And once I took that step, my destiny took a step toward me. I received a $12,000 scholarship for my first semester. Miraculously, my job was willing to decrease my hours and keep me at the same pay rate. Doors opened for me that I could not have planned or anticipated. As I took that step forward following my inner compass, more was revealed. Cerato often requires a leap of faith and an act of trust. As Dr. Martin Luther King Jr. once said, "Faith is taking the first step, even when you don't see the whole staircase." [19]

Disconnect between what we feel and what we see creates anxiety. Cerato is a great flower essence if you're feeling indecisive, especially when your heart is telling you one thing but your mind is telling you something different. It's also a flower essence to use whenever your mind is clouded with a lot of advice from other people. When we receive too much input, we start to look for answers outside of ourselves—we ask our friends what we should do or what they think about the situation, we research online, we seek guidance from our mentors. But at the end of the day, we know the truth when we're standing in it. We feel it in our bones.

Cerato reminds me of the stories of the goddess Osun. Osun wanders from village to village, asking everyone what she should do. She receives great—but conflicting—advice. At the end of the day, she decides not to follow anyone

19. Martin Luther King Jr. Quotes", *Goodreads* website. https://www.goodreads.com/quotes/16312-faith-is-taking-the-first-step-even-when-you-can-t.

but her own heart. That's Cerato—the ability to listen to our inner voice, trust our inner wisdom, and have the courage to stand behind it.

Mugwort: Listen to Your Dreams—While all flower essence will affect our dream life, Mugwort plays a special role in dream recall and understanding. When I work with clients, I don't advise them to run out to buy a dream dictionary. Why? Our dreams are personal and draw on associations from our own lives. Think of your dreams as a good friend with a special handshake. You and your dreams have a shared secret language of symbol, myth, and metaphor. And like a good friend, assume that the dream is coming to share something that you don't already know consciously, to offer a new perspective, and to further your evolution.[20]

Even the most disturbing dreams may be simply trying to get your attention. Bring patience, compassion, and a willingness to listen. The more you work with your dreams, the more you will be able to develop systems and a language that work for you.

Soul Medicine Practice: Dream Catching

The following tips will help you cultivate a lasting relationship with your dream life while working with flower essences, and mugwort flower essence in particular.

Keep a Dream Journal

Buy or create a dream journal that you can keep next to your bed, along with a pen. If necessary, it may also be helpful to have a small light or candle if you typically wake up in a dark room. The journal should be exclusively for dreams. It may be helpful to organize your journal in such a way that there is space on one side to record your dream, and another side to record your associations, translations, and interpretations as you move through your day. If writing is not your thing, using the Voice Memo app on your phone is another way to capture the dream while it is still fresh. There are also some great (free) apps that will type your words as you speak. There is no right or wrong way to create a dream journal, as long as it works for you.

---

20. Robert A. Johnson, *Inner Work: Using Dreams and Active Imagination for Personal Growth* (New York: HarperOne, 2009), page.

Record the Dream

Now that you have a dream journal, the next step is recording the dream. Catching a dream is a bit like catching dew in the morning before it starts to evaporate. Dreaming engages your yin states of awareness and perception, so the more you move and activate your yang physiology (metabolism, logical thinking), the less you will be able to remember. Ideally, record your dream as soon as you wake up. If you wake up in the middle of the night with a dream, it's best to record it at that moment instead of waiting until morning. There may be times when your memory of a dream is triggered by a life event. In those cases, record what you remember and what triggered it as soon as possible, and then add it to your dream journal at a later time.

Give It a Title

Giving your dream a title is a great way to summarize the story of the dream until you have time to record full details. It is similar to television sitcom episodes that have a title (for example: "The One Where She Loses Her Keys," or "The Fork in the Road"). You'll be surprised at how much a title can gather up key events or themes of the dream until you're able to write down the details. Sometimes even just coming up with a title for the dream will give insight into its meaning and message.

Record the Emotions

If a dream evokes a feeling or felt sense (such as shock, fear, elation, a pit in your stomach) record that as well. You can work with the feeling of the dream just as effectively as working with the details and events of a dream.

Tune In to One Image

Dreams, just like life, are holographic. In a holographic view, essential meaning of the whole is encoded into each small piece of the original.[21] This means that any one symbol or image from the dream can be encoded in the message of the entire dream. Tune in to an image that feels alive, awake, or particularly

---

21. Pam Montgomery, *Plant Spirit Healing: A Guide to Working with Plant Consciousness* (Rochester, VT: Bear & Co., 2008), 13.

vibrant or luminous. Jot down as many details as you can while attuning your inner focus to that image.

Establish Ritual

It can often be helpful to create a ritual around your dream life to establish a container or vessel for this level of soul work. Examples include going to sleep with a question written on a piece of paper under your pillow, or starting each day by lighting a candle and writing for an amount of time. Many of us have busy schedules that require us to jump out of bed and get going right away. In those cases, committing to dream journaling on the new or full moon, a specific day of the week or month (for example, every Monday, the seventh of each month, and so on) can be a helpful way to make space for your dreams. Remember to stay open to dreams that may come at other times with their own intentions and messages.

Embodied Practice: Balasana (Child's Pose)

Affirmation: I take time to listen

Begin by kneeling on the ground. Gently hinge at the waist to fold over your legs, drawing your hips toward your heels. If this is uncomfortable, place a block or folded blanket between your butt and your heels. Extend your arms on the ground in front of you as you rest your forehead on the floor or a block. Find ease in the pose, adjusting into a position that is most comfortable for your body.

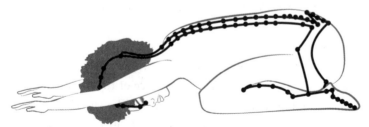

Pictured with the Bladder Meridian

Take several deep breaths as you listen from within. Close your eyes, turn your senses inward, and repeat the affirmation: *I take time to listen.*

Soul Lesson 3: You Are Ancient

"A people without knowledge of their past history,
origin and culture is like a tree without roots."
—*Marcus Garvey*

If you observe a bean sprouting in a glass bowl, you will see that before it rises to break through the soil, its roots sink down to anchor the plant firmly in place. This beautiful moment in nature embodies the West African principle of *Sankofa*, which means that to know where you are going, you have to know where you've been. The popular Adinkra symbol depicts a bird who flies forward while looking backward to see behind it.

In African and many Indigenous spiritual systems, we know that our ancestors are guiding and watching over us. It is our responsibility to honor their legacy by acting in good character and achieving our destiny, and they are there to help us along the way. Water is poured as libation to these benevolent ancestors and acts as a conduit between worlds. The Water element connects us to our physical and spiritual roots and the collective wisdom that comes from our ancestors, our family history, and our past experiences. When we delve into the past to understand who we are and where we are going, we call on the wisdom of Water. Our ancestry, the genealogical imprint in our DNA and nervous system, and our personal and collective history are embodied in the Water element. This wisdom and communion helps us transform the Water element's fear, anxiety, and uncertainty into trust, perseverance, and courage.

In Chinese Medicine, *jing* refers to the essences inherited from our parents. Whenever there are hereditary illnesses passed down through the family tree, we are looking at a manifestation of jing. Every time we go to a doctor's appointment and complete an intake form about our family's medical history, we are considering our jing. The Water element connects us to our biological, emotional, and spiritual inheritance. Water holds the ancestral seed passed from one generation to the next.

Humans have a long ancestral history of using stories and symbols to share spiritual wisdom. Today, we can look at popular movies, shows, and songs that carry the archetypal truths a culture is trying to integrate. It's fascinating stuff, and Joseph Campbell's work on the power of myth goes into great detail about how these myths reflect and affect culture.[22] The exploration of personal and collective myths is also a strategy used in Jungian depth psychology. The Water element helps us to access and relate to the stories in our collective human consciousness.

I tend to learn best from animated movies, superhero comics, and musicals, but that's just me. Whenever I am obsessed to the point of uncontrollable binge-watching or reading, I know I have tapped into a character or story that has symbolic meaning in my life. My niece, a wise teenager, says that her generation calls this phenomenon "kinning." Popular especially in anime culture, kinning involves relating to a character so much that you develop a psychic bond. It can include dressing like the character or in extreme cases, believing you *are* the character as you take on their behaviors and mannerisms. When life imitates art in this way, the Water element is certainly involved.

The movie *Frozen 2* is a great archetypal story of the Water element that also illustrates the soul messages of Joshua Tree and Saguaro. In Disney's *Frozen*, we meet Elsa, a princess with the magical power to create ice and snow (hello, Water element!). In the 2019 sequel, Elsa is guided on a journey to the River of Ahtohallan, the river that her deceased mother told her holds the history of the past. In psychology, we would say that this river holds the collective unconsciousness. In metaphysics, this river represents the Akashic record. If you're a *Game of Thrones* fan, we could say this river is like the three-eyed raven—it knows everything that ever was, is, and could be. The river calls to Elsa in a mysterious, haunting voice, and Elsa decides to journey into the unknown to discover its source.

Throughout *Frozen 2*, the phrase "water has memory" is a recurring theme. Elsa learns from the waters, revealed as images literally frozen in time. During her quest, Elsa discovers that her magical powers come from her mother's people, the Nuthuldran tribe, who are the indigenous inhabitants of the enchanted forest. She also learns that her grandfather betrayed the Nuthuldran people and created a dam to block their access to magic. Not only that, she sees an image of her grandfather violently slaying the peaceful leader of the Nuthuldran tribe while in prayer.

---

22. Joseph Campbell, Bill D. Moyers, and Betty S. Flowers, *The Power of Myth* (Saint Louis, MO: Turtleback Books, 2012).

Elsa bears the responsibility of restoring the integrity of her family line by cleaning up this negative karma. The blessings of her lineage must be balanced by righting the trauma and violence that are also part of her lineage in order for her to truly stand in her magic. The Water element helps us explore both the gifts that come from our lineage, as well as the curses. Water invites us to ask: How do we live into the blessings and the gifts of our family line? How do we acknowledge the crisis and the trauma, and *move it forward?* How do these lessons affect or inform our destiny? To answer these questions requires the humble awareness of the miracle of events that conspired for us to be who we are, in this time and place.

Frozen 2 is a perfect example of life imitating art, and art imitating life. Ancestral magic, generational legacies, mystery, hidden truths, fear, trust, and diving into the unknown are key themes in the film, and signatures of the Water element. This movie also emerges at the same time as a growing conversation about the legacy and trauma that the United States is built on, and the unhealed wounds beginning to emerge from the shadows of the American psyche.

Water has memory. Dr. Masaru Emoto's work is an incredible example of how water records our thoughts and intentions. In his studies, he viewed the difference between water crystals that have been charged with positive words (such as love, joy, or peace) or negative expressions (such as hate, guilt, or pain).[23] The crystals from water charged with positive words are beautifully symmetrical and harmonious, while those charged with negative words appear fragmented and chaotic.

Water has memory, a fact that has been true for lifetimes. African Diasporic traditions use water to communicate with ancestors through pouring libation. Ceremonies, rituals, celebrations, and gatherings all begin with libation, a practice of evoking the memory of those who have transcended to the spiritual realm and are available for support and guidance. The Family Constellation Healing System, developed by Bert Hellinger in the 1990s, is another healing modality that supports this aspect of the Water element. Family Constellations, also known as Systemic Constellations, was developed after Hellinger spent extensive time learning from the cultural and spiritual

---

23. Masaru Emoto, *The Miracle of Water* (New York: Atria Books, 2011).

practices of the Zulu peoples of southern Africa. Family Constellation facil-itators guide participants in recognizing outdated agreements, unhealthy dynamics, and unrevealed secrets within the family history. It is a powerful and profound practice that I liken to "acupuncture on the family tree."

When I shared my experience with Family Constellations with my sister-in-love,[24] an initiate of Yemonja in the Lucumi tradition, she pointed out the similarities between Hellinger's work and a *misa*. A misa is an investigative ceremony in which elders consult ancestors and other spiritual guides for insight into how the client can reach their fullest potential.[25] Just as in a Fam-ily Constellation, family secrets and blessings are discovered. Members in the circle may embody the energies of folks who are not physically present but have insight or information that can shift the dynamics of the client's situa-tion. The Water element supports our connection to the streams of awareness that bridge individual and collective consciousness.

We not only receive the gifts, blessings and guidance of our ancestors. The wounds and trauma experienced by our ancestors also live on through our nervous system. When working with the Water element, we are invited to heal these wounds, receive our blessings, and refresh our family tree for future generations. The Water element teaches us how to honor the wisdom that came before us, and the shoulders we stand on.

Reflection Questions

What is your legacy? Take a moment to reflect on the following questions in your journal:

+ What are your family's origins? How did you come to be here, now?
+ What gifts and traits have you inherited from your parents? From your grandparents? From your great-grandparents?
+ What is your relationship with your ancestors? What are their names?
+ What, if any, are the wounds that keep you from connecting to your ancestral lineage?

---

24. The term "sister-in-love" is a much easier, and more accurate way to describe the relationship with my ex-husband's brother's wife.

25. Ava Tiye Kinsey, conversation with the author, September 2021.

* What, if any, grievances from your family line need to be reconciled?
* What positive memories define your relationship with your family?

Flower Essences for Your Ancient Connection

The flower essences that support our ability to connect to our past are:

* Joshua Tree for matrilineal lessons and blessings
* Saguaro for patrilineal lessons and blessings
* Lilac for remembering the good

Joshua Tree and Saguaro: Ancestral Lessons and Blessings—Joshua Tree and Saguaro are closely related essences that together help us to explore our generational wounds, blessings, and lessons. Both are cactus flowers that survive the high temperatures of a desert climate. However, saguaro blooms in the sun, while Joshua tree is a night blooming moon flower. As is fitting with Yin and Yang theory, Saguaro helps us to explore our relationship with our male ancestors and patrilineal line, while Joshua Tree opens the door to our female ancestors and matrilineal line.

Saguaro and Joshua Tree are flower essences that help to awaken the memories, lessons, and blessings of our ancestors. In their own ways, both open the door to intergenerational healing and exploration. They often help us attract the resources—like the essences and practices mentioned above—to dive even deeper. They work well together and individually. Joshua Tree supports us as we acknowledge our family history and cultural connections but still need to carve a new path that is authentic to our individual gifts. It also helps us to witness, and if necessary, break from unhealthy dynamics. When dysfunctional or problematic beliefs threaten to keep us from evolving forward, Joshua Tree flower essence brings healing and a new perspective. It helps us uncover dysfunctional family beliefs, secrets, and shame. Saguaro moves in the opposite direction by helping us to build a stronger connection to the wisdom, cultural traditions, and authority of living and deceased elders. It is especially helpful if we have distain, distrust, or disconnection from our roots. Both flower essences support us as we chart a path that brings renewal to the whole family tree.

Lilac: Remember the Good—Lilac helps us to remember the experiences in this lifetime that have profoundly touched our soul or inspired us. Lilac is one of my favorite remedies to turn to when an aspect of our soul memory is lacking. Clinically, I've found this flower very healing and useful when someone is going through a period of intense inner work. This can be through spiritual training or practice that requires us to look closely at our faults or mistakes. This can also be due to therapy or counseling, which often calls us to dig into painful memories of the past in order to understand our current situation. Exploring early childhood wounds in individual therapy or exploring the root of the breakdown of a relationship in couples' therapy can lead us into Water's depths. The experience can be intensely painful as the repressed memories resurface, bringing with them tides of emotional and even physical discomfort. Lilac serves as a benevolent gift to help us recall the good memories that were also suppressed.

Lilac flower essence reminds me of a moment in *Eternal Sunshine of the Spotless Mind*. In this quirky sci-fi movie, Jim Carrey's character is having the memory of his relationship-gone-sour erased. The memories at the beginning of the erasure process—the most recent—are the most painful. However, as he fast-rewinds through time to the beginning of the relationship, he finds memories that he had long forgotten: intimate moments, a laugh, a touch. These moments appear like clips from a movie in his mind, very much the same way Lilac gently calls memories to the surface of our awareness.

And just like in the movie, we often find that painful memories are more accessible than pleasant ones. They call our attention because they are trying to teach us something. Lilac supports us in remembering the sacred, the beautiful, the inspiring moments and the magic they brought to our lives. In their quiet way, those moments also have something important to teach us.

I used Lilac flower essence when I was going through the most challenging moments of my divorce. My memories of the relationship were full of anger and rage, which was necessary to move forward. Without the righteous indignation and anger of the Wood element (explored in the next chapter), I would have likely stayed in unhealthy relationship patterns. The anger served a purpose, but I could not let that same rage run our mediation sessions. We were trying to make a co-parenting agreement that worked for everyone. Lilac helped me to remember the sweeter moments buried beneath the anger and hurt, and it helped me to navigate the challenging moments with my love forces and humanity intact. Lilac surfaced memories that reminded me, "there is also great love here."

Lilac flower essence helps us to integrate those beautiful memories, teaching us that our experiences cannot be classified in black and white terms—right or wrong, good or bad. Instead, we come to understand that our experiences are just like the primordial forces of yin and yang—both light and dark, forever dancing together and weaving the rich, colorful tapestry of our lives.

Embodied Practice: Parsvottanasana (Pyramid Pose)

Affirmation: I take time to remember

From a standing position, take a large step three to five feet forward. Bring your heels into one line. Face your front toes forward, and angle your back foot to your comfort (at around 45 degrees). Square your hips forward in the direction of your front toes, like shining two headlight beams in the direction you are going. Gently hinge at the hips to bring your chest toward your front knee. Reach your hands in front of you to grasp your ankle or shin, or to rest on blocks. Bend your knees slightly if the stretch along your hamstrings and back (your Water meridians) is too intense. Notice that you are embodying the principle of Sankofa: as you step forward, you can see behind you.

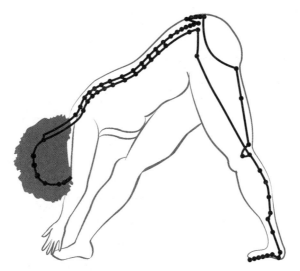

Pictured with the Bladder Meridian

Imagine that you are a triangle, in the form of an ancient pyramid. The triangle shape represents the past, present, and the future. Acknowledge that all three are with you in this moment as you repeat the affirmation: *I take time to remember.*

Hold the pose for a few moments, and then repeat with the opposite foot forward. In your journal, record any insights or understandings that emerge.

Music Is Medicine: Playlist for the Water Element

Your Water element playlist will include music that helps you feel calm, serene, introspective, and connected to your power. Your playlist may also evoke courage, stability, and perseverance. Below are some favorites on my list that express the archetypal signatures and sounds of the Water element. See the resources section at the end of this book to find links to playlists generated by myself and students!

"Silence Is the Way" by Miles Davis & Robert Glasper featuring Laura Mvula
Album: The Dreaming Room, Sony Music Entertainment, 2016

I love this jazzy hip-hopera! The Water element governs our sense of hearing and listening. Try this: close your eyes and see if you can identify the quietest sound in the room. Listen underneath the most obvious sounds (here in NYC, there are plenty!) and tune in. Notice how that attentiveness brings you fully present to the here and now? That's the gift of Water: a stillness and presence that allows us to transmute fear into cautious awareness of our environment. Indeed, the Water element invites us to listen to silence.

"River" by Ibeyi
Album: Ibeyi, XL Recordings, 2014

From baptism to libation, Water is used across religions as a conduit between worlds. Water draws us in to our depths. The energetic direction of water is downward, as water always seeks the deepest level. Water surrenders to gravity, descending down…down…down—just like the cadence of this praise song. Soothing, healing, yielding, cleansing, the Water element is a powerful force of healing and spiritual cleansing.

"Dark Side of the Moon" by Lil Wayne featuring Nicki Minaj
Album: *Tha Carter V, Young Money/Republic, 2018*

This soulful duet is written almost entirely in the language of the Water element—in metaphor and symbols. The Water element is associated with the moon and her intuitive, reflective power. The Water element brings us deep within ourselves, where we can access our intuition. The moon is also associated with our lunar state of consciousness, and our ability to access our alpha, delta, and theta states of awareness and perception.

"Same Ol' Mistakes" by Rihanna
Album: *Anti, Westbury Road/Roc Nation, 2016*

Oooh. I've been there, Riri! It's amazing how knowing better doesn't mean we'll actually *do* better. That's because the Water element corresponds to the subconscious mind, and the shadowy aspects of our soul that control our behavior when we least expect it. That's why, try as we might, we find ourselves being held in the spell of people, places, and experiences that we can't walk away from. The Water element's gravity bounds us to our mistakes until we surrender to its depths. This song's low, crawling tones evoke the depth and shadow that are home to the Water element's treasures.

"Weary" by Solange
Album: *A Seat at the Table, Saint/Columbia Records, 2016*

Oh Solange, you nailed it with this song! With all the political happenings and the ways of the world, many of us are feeling that weariness! The Water element teaches us to retreat and replenish our inner reserves. If you're feeling burned out, less inclined to go out and party, or unmotivated to take on new projects, the Water element is having her way with you.

Magic by Coldplay
Album: Ghost Stories, Parlophone/Atlantic Records, 2014

The Water element governs the part of us that is cosmic, mystical, and magical. The deep study of philosophical ideas or history, metaphysical wisdom or the mystery sciences is in the realm of the Water element.

"I Put a Spell on You" by Alice Smith
Album: NINA REVISITED: A Tribute to Nina Simone,
RCA Records, 2015

On the subject of magic, Alice Smith's rendition of this Nina Simone classic is utterly spellbinding. The Water element corresponds to the archetype of the Goddess who governs the when and how of manifesting our intentions. She shows up across cultures as the oceanic goddesses of creation and magic: Yemoja of the Ifa tradition, Auset of Kemetic mythology, Sedna of the Inuit peoples, Amphitrite of the Greek pantheon, and La Sirene of Voodun faith.

"Astronomy (8th Light)" by Black Star
Album: Mos Def and Talib Kweli are Black Star,
Rawkus/Priority/EMI/MCA, 1998

Though we often associate water with shades of blue, the Water element in Chinese Medicine is classically associated with a dark, blue-black color. Black draws itself within, evoking the introspective, mysterious power of the Water element. I love Black Star's ode to blackness in Astronomy (the 8th Light).

"Legacy" by Jay-Z featuring Blue Ivy
Album: 4:44, Roc Nation, 2017

I would consider almost the entire 4:44 album a tribute to the Water element, with its strong head nod to family, roots, and lineage. In "Legacy," Jay calls into question the lessons that were passed down through his family tree. The Water element helps us do exactly that—examine the earliest beliefs about love, relationships, and wealth that we inherited from our family of origin. We can then create a new branch that refreshes our family tree.

My Jamaica by Nakeeba Amaniyea featuring Sister Carol
Independent Single, Blakwater House Studio, 2020

Speaking of legacy, in "My Jamaica" songbird and lyricist Nakeeba picks up the creative torch from reggae legend "Mother Culture" Sister Carol. The Water element teaches us how to understand where we come from in order to understand where we're going. In this mother-daughter duet, we witness a new branch blooming on a family tree with deep cultural roots.

"Comes to Light (everything)" by Jill Scott
Album: Golden Moments, *Hidden Beach Recordings*, 2015

After the winter solstice, the deepest expression of yin, the days begin to get longer as the light returns. The Water element represents that turning point in nature and in our psyche. Water introduces us to our shadow—the unilluminated, unintegrated parts of our personality. Water challenges us to withstand the darkness (the quiet, the stillness, and sometimes even the chaos) while trusting that the light will return. Water gives us the faith that after even the darkest night, we can trust that there will be light—insight, clarity, and healing.

"I Don't Get Tired (#IDGT)" Kevin Gates featuring August Alsina
Album: Luca Brasi 2, *Bread Winners Association/Atlantic*, 2014

If you've got six jobs, you *should* be tired. This speaks to the tenacity, perseverance and sheer will that are signatures of Water. The Water element helps us when we're in either side of burnout, even in that phase of being so charged up that we don't know we're doing too much. The Water element helps us cue in to our body's true need for rest and replenishing our hearts after we've overextended ourselves. It's the perfect remedy when you feel like you have so much to do, there's no way you can take a break.

"Just Like Water (Live)" by Ms. Lauryn Hill
Album: MTV Unplugged No. 2.0, *Columbia Records*, 2002

This playlist wouldn't be complete without Lauryn's literal ode to the metaphorical power of Water. (Lauren's gravelly voice is also characteristic of those with a strong constitutional Water element). I love this song because when we have a healthy relationship with abundance, we can easily express gratitude for all the blessings we have. We know deeply and instinctively that we have more than enough … and can find our flow.

Water in Practice: Making a Prayer Board

A favorite activity to embrace the gifts of the Water element is making a prayer board. A prayer board is very similar to a vision board, and both are powerful tools for manifesting our desires. But there's some very key differences between the two. A prayer board is like a dreamscape. You use intuition, images, symbols, poetry, and song lyrics. While making a prayer board, stay tuned to what speaks to you, what you're drawn to, and what inspires you without putting a whole lot of thought into why and what it means. We're not going for logic here. Here are some key differences that make prayer boards unique:

1. **Intention**

   Vision boards focus on what you want to achieve or acquire (e.g., a promotion at work, a vacation abroad, a car, etc.) and are best created when you can clearly see what you want—hence the name. A prayer board focuses on who you want to become and what you want to feel. So rather than envisioning a promotion, you might include symbols that remind you to stand in your power and stand up for your worth. Instead of a hot vacay destination, your board might tap into feelings of relaxation, serenity, or even adventure. The point is *why*, not the *what*.

2. **Openness**

   A vision board focuses on a specific goal, e.g., "I want to raise $30,000." Prayer boards are wonderful because we don't always know the exact thing we need. I know want to feel abundant, but it may manifest in different ways. The Water element helps me trust the forces that walk with me to bring that abundance to me in a way that is in my highest and best interest. A prayer board holds the feeling of your intention but allows for many ways of manifestation. It is like saying "this or something better" at the end of a prayer: it keeps us from limiting our expectations to what we already know to be possible. A prayer board allows space for the expansiveness of the universe to flood us with insight, solutions, and opportunities beyond what we might have imagined. We surrender what we think we want for our lives to receive the abundance that is already effortlessly flowing our way.

For example, one of my goals this year is to increase my public speaking engagements. Instead of using the names of specific places where I'd like to present, I am using a microphone so that I can attract the right opportunities. I might end up somewhere I'd never have thought to explore, and I'm open to the right workings of a universe that has never steered me wrong. An added bonus is that the symbol reminds me to speak my truth, which will serve me not only in my career but in all my relationships.

3. Language

A vision board often has affirmations and words that act as reminders of what to do or how to act. It is a message to your will, to influence your conscious actions and beliefs. Prayer boards use language as reminders from your highest self to your subconscious mind. Poems, prayers, and passages from sacred texts work nicely amid the symbolic images of a prayer board. Lyrics from songs that we wake up with in the morning often make for great Prayer Board material. Last year, I worked with the simple prayer "let there be light"— equally inspired by Genesis 1:3 and the 2006 song by Nas. It was my prayer to bring healing to my estranged relationships, to illuminate my shadowy parts, and to bring insight during times of uncertainty.

4. Images

A vision board has images of what you specifically want to manifest; anyone else looking at your vision board could pretty much know what you're working on. A prayer board has images that are highly symbolic, personal, and archetypal. It looks and feels like a dream. Images of actual people are replaced with artistic or silhouetted forms. Symbols of nature appear as metaphors for the qualities we want to embody. Goddesses, Orisha, and astrological symbols remind us of who we are becoming: the adventurer, the nurturer, the healer, the lover, the warrior. When I am planning to start my prayer board,

I spend a week or two noticing and collecting the images that pop on my social media feeds that strike a chord.

5. Intuition and Felt Sense

Both vision and prayer board-making are highly creative, intuitive processes. Prayer boards also rely on inner sensing—an inner click, feeling, or sensation that we get when something is right for us, even when we don't consciously know why. (It's very similar to the sense we get when something is wrong or off that we can't put a finger on, but in the opposite direction!) This means that while making a prayer board, there might be images or symbols that deeply resonate with you but you can't articulate why in a coherent way. They just *feel* right and something in your body "leans in."

Case in point: Five years ago, I felt drawn to yoga and chakra images. I had no idea why, especially since my yoga practice over the past few years had been spotty at best. But there I was, attracted to image after image. A vinyasa sun salutation found its way to the bottom of my board. A wild chakra lady covered the right corner. And six months later, beyond all logic and reason, I found myself on a plane to Costa Rica for an intensive, three-week yoga teacher training. It was not something I had ever intended to do, but the doors opened so effortlessly that I couldn't help but walk through.

Through the process of making a prayer board, you can practice your skills trusting your intuition, following your inner compass, and opening yourself to divine guidance.

Chapter 4
Marching Wood

The image of the sprout is a guiding metaphor for the Wood element in our souls. This sprout does not ask for its share of the sun; it just grows instinctively toward the light. The Wood element teaches us how to grow and expand. We go after what we need to actualize our greatness without the need for permission or validation.

Wood Element Signatures

We recognize the archetypal qualities of the Wood element in the following signatures:

- Season: Spring
- Phase: Sprout
- Color: Green
- Energetic: Rises qi
- Core Emotion: Anger
- Sound: Shouting
- Meridians: Liver and Gallbladder

Season: Spring

We encounter the Wood element when we see the first buds of nature sprouting. All winter long, those seeds have been deep in the ground, gathering the strength they need for that defining moment when they must break open and push through the soil. There is movement originating out of stillness, and a push forward with clear purpose and direction.

Phase: Sprout

Like the sprout as it emerges from under ground, the Wood element represents the beginning phase and supports us whenever we are starting something new. It is associated with sunrise, and the hope inspired by the dawn of a new day. When the Wood element awakens in the earliest days of spring, the life force of nature begins to stir beneath the ground.

The beginning of something, the initiation, marks a first step toward change. The *I Ching*, the divination text of ancient China, describes the awakening life force in the third hexagram: Thunder beneath the Water. These rumblings—this stirring of the life force in early February—is what wakes up our wise old groundhog and sends her above ground after her deep sleep of winter. The third hexagram, *chun*, is translated as "difficulty in the beginning" because, well, it *is* difficult in the early stages of emerging change.

The rumblings of the Wood element take many forms. Sometimes they show up as discontent, boredom, or discomfort, inspiring us a step into a new career. Sometimes the rumblings are frustration and impatience, asking us to initiate change in our relationships. Sometimes the rumblings are revolutionary and inspire us to step into leadership in our communities. The rumblings awaken us from illusion, ignorance, and slumber, and invite us to take a stand for who we are and what we hold valuable.

Color: Green

In Classical Five Element acupuncture, the color of the Wood element is green. We experience this green when we look at the variations of color in a field of grass and the brilliant forest canopy in the spring. Green is also found in moss and any kind of chlorophyll, the "blood" of the plant world. We use phrases like "green with envy" to describe someone whose Wood element is negatively comparing them to another person. Bringing green plants into any space will bring the Wood element's qualities of liveliness, grace, and ease into the room.

Energetic: Rises Qi

Wood rises the qi. The true intention of anger is change; it is the energy required to evolve something or move it forward. What happens when the upward motion of change and evolution gets obstructed? It does one of two things: it pushes harder until it explodes so that it can continue its intended upward trajectory. Or, it gets tired of pushing upward and sinks downward, becoming a form of depression or resignation. Variations of anger include frustration, agitation, irritability, resentment, hostility, bitterness, exasperation, annoyance, and rage. When balanced, the Wood element gifts us with a sense of contentment and ease. Feeling *irie*, the Rastafarian word that loosely translates as "all is well, no worries" perfectly describes the feeling of a healthy Wood element.

Core Emotion: Anger

Anger is the core emotion associated with the Wood element, having an upward momentum that raises the qi. If we consider that symbolic sprout, we get a good picture of what we mean by the power of the Wood element. Gravity is the force that holds everything to the earth—from cars and skyscrapers to mountains and oceans. Gravity keeps everything from floating up into space; it's that strong. And yet, a tiny little sprout manages to push against the force of gravity as it reaches toward the sky. Can you imagine what would happen if that sprout didn't have the incredible push to break through the to the other side? It would stay a seed forever. Any plant that is not willfully looking for the sun or the nutrients it needs to thrive is not going to live very long. And when we don't actively get what we need and deserve, the Wood element in us calls for our attention. This upward, forceful energy is the gift of the Wood element.

Often the first thing we think of when we hear the word *anger* is conflict, or even violence. Yet, the Wood element teaches us that conflict is necessary for anything to evolve. Conflict is an opportunity to reconcile opposing points of view and to find win-win solutions that work for everyone involved. Conflict also offers the opportunity to reconcile what was and has always been with what is possible for the future. Anger is a signal that something needs to change. We need force and need power to move toward change—just as the sprout needs force and power to resist the pull of gravity.

In Chinese Medicine, one of the most famous herbal formulas is called *xiao yao san*, translated as "the free and easy wanderer." When in harmony, the Wood element enables us to move through our lives with freedom and ease, and no fear of being harmed. The Wood element is expressed through benevolence, and knowing that we can get what we need, without taking from or exploiting anyone else. When violated, the Wood element becomes a warrior for justice. Whether it's social justice, or personal justice, the Wood element asserts that we *all* have the right to live with freedom and ease. The Wood element also teaches us how to respond with righteous indignation or anger when that right is violated. Through the Wood element, we learn to assert our boundaries and fight for equity and respect. It is the revolutionary force that pushes against gravity to create new paradigms. The upward energy of the Wood element is a movement toward life.

Listed below are a few variations of emotions that may be evoked with the upward trajectory of the Wood element is compromised:

Anger	Resentment	Belligerence	Frustration
Envy	Sarcasm	Annoyance	Agitation
Aggravation	Aggression	Irritability	Bitterness
Outrage	Hostility	Hopelessness/ Resignation	Intimidation

Sound: Shouting

The sound of the Wood element in a person's voice conveys focused intention and direction. Have you ever talked to someone whose words were so forceful and clear that you almost wanted to duck? That's the Wood element! Classically, a characteristically Wood voice is called *shouting*, which relates more to its quality—pointed and direct—than to its actual volume. A shouting voice can project clearly, which is why it bodes well for public speakers and others who lead with their voice. Shouting can also sound clipped or abrupt, something you can hear in an exaggerated way when you hold your breath and say, "The grass is always greener."

In music, we evoke the energy of the Wood element with songs whose lyrics inspire us to decisive action. Music with a strong staccato rhythm, and with an upward or climbing melody, is also evocative of the Wood element. My Wood element playlist includes songs that inspire me to action and give me a confidence boost.

Meridians: Liver and Gallbladder

The organs associated with the Wood element are the Liver and Gallbladder. The Liver meridian begins at the inner corner of the big toe nail, travels along the top of the foot, along the inner leg through the groin, around the genitals, and terminates near the diaphragm. An inner branch of this channel ascends through the throat, making it a powerful channel to regulate our creative expression. [**Figure 4.1**] There are also great pressure points along the channel that create ease and flow in the menstrual cycle. The Gallbladder meridian starts at the outer corner of the eye, and then zig zags across the side of the head before wandering back and forth along the side of the body. [**Figure 4.2**] It's no surprise that indecisiveness, a pattern of the Wood element, is expressed in the indirect, alternating path of this meridian. When we're gearing up to fight—psychologically or physically—these two meridians get congested and create neck and shoulder tension. We may also experience indigestion, reproductive issues, irregular cycles, or migraines when internalizing the Wood

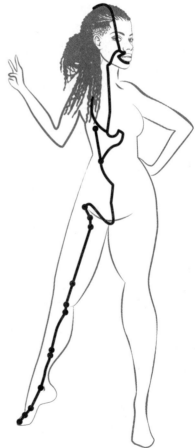

4.1 Liver Meridian

element's propensity for tension and conflict. Symptoms that direct us to the Wood meridians include:

- Neck and shoulder tension
- Upper back pain
- Menstrual problems (especially heavy or painful periods)
- Muscle cramps and spasms
- Emotional holding in the hips and groins
- Migraines
- Indigestion
- Constipation

In yoga practice, postures that evoke the power of the Wood element include all warrior poses, especially when practiced with affirmations of power and assertiveness. These postures also activate the Wood element meridians that course along the inner and outer legs. Any posture or breathing exercise that strengthens the core abdominal muscles or fires up the solar plexus benefits the Wood element, as do hip openers that release stored anger and hurt that may not have been expressed. Finally, lengthening, flowing movement helps us to embody the flexibility that the Wood element gifts us.

The Wood element is called "the general" because it has the vision along with the power and strategy to execute a plan. What does a war general do in times of peace? It goes out to explore "new" lands, something that does not work out well for those of us on the receiving side of that exploration, because the drive to conquer and ruthlessly dominate is part of the shadow consciousness of the Wood element. The Wood element's impulses for exploration, self-actualization, and winning at all costs are deeply embodied in the mythos of the Western world, with both negative and positive expressions.

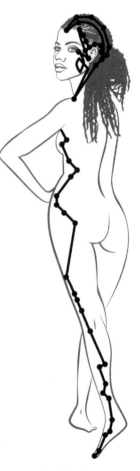

4.2 Gallbladder Meridian

The Wood element is associated with youth and adolescence, especially the teenage phase. A great way to get a sense of the Wood archetype is to envision a badass, rebellious teenager who knows what they want—freedom! Independence! Autonomy! In this natural stage in their development, teenagers want respect for their unique opinions and perspectives. The Wood element also expresses itself as impulsiveness and defensiveness, both of which are typical teenage qualities as they learn how to assert their vision, and to define themselves. This usually means pushing against the gravity of their family's values, traditions, and support. They say things like, "Don't help me," "Don't tell me what to do," and "I can do it myself," and get angry if they feel controlled or powerless. But the success of Wood is rooted in the Water element's wisdom. Teenagers, as awesome as they are, lack the wisdom of experience and need guidance from wise elders. The result? Conflict, Wood element style!

When allowed to grow toward the sun, the Wood element brings innovation, creativity, new opportunities, and a fresh perspective. During the 2021 presidential inauguration, teen phenomenon Amanda Gorman perfectly exemplified the Wood element's ability to bring light to a dark time. In the midst of racial conflict, the youngest inaugural poet in US history fearlessly called out America's struggle and presented a new vision. Her poem, "The Hill We Climb," ends with a call for the bravery to see the light of a new dawn—all Wood element signatures.[26] I can only imagine the unshakable courage it must have taken for this young Black teen to stand in front of the world and speak eloquently on the Capitol steps—the same steps that two weeks before had been under siege by protestors that too closely resembled a lynch mob. When we embody the Wood element, we embody this tremendous bravery, tremendous vision, and tremendous possibility.

Soul Lesson 1: Anger=Change

Usually when people are sad, they don't do anything. They just cry over their condition. But when they get angry, they bring about a change.
—*Malcolm X*

Take a moment to think about the last time you were really angry. I'm not talking about your run-of-the-mill irritation at someone cutting you off.

---

26. Amanda Gorman, *The Hill We Climb: Poems* (New York: Viking Children's Books, 2021).

Instead, try to remember a moment you felt deeply affected by a conflict with someone you care about.

What did you do in that moment? How did it feel in your body? How did you respond, and were you satisfied with the outcome? In fact—was there even an outcome? Did anything change because of your anger?

Remember that flower growing instinctively toward the sun? It's not saying, "excuse me, other flowers, do you mind if I reach for the light?" Or, "Oops, sorry, I didn't mean to take up too much light. My bad!" Nope, that little sprout just goes for it without asking for permission, validation, or forgiveness. The Wood element supports the aspect of ourselves that is also striving and going for the sun, trying to live our best life. Anger is the natural, organic, and appropriate response to being blocked from the sun. When we are blocked, one of two things will happen: we either explode with enough force to continue moving forward, or we give up and sink back into the soil.

One of my favorite movies to illustrate this aspect of the Wood element in action is the 2003 movie *Anger Management* starring Jack Nicholson and Adam Sandler. The movie was released in the spring of that year—you guessed it, right on time for the Wood element season! In it, Jack Nicholson's character explains:

> There are two kinds of angry people: explosive and implosive. Explosive is the kind of individual that you see screaming at the cashier for not taking their coupons [...]
>
> Implosive is the cashier who remains quiet day after day, and finally shoots everyone in the store.[27]

Take a look at the anger trigger you previously identified. Did you implode, holding in your feelings and tension in your body? Or did you explode, letting everyone know exactly where they could go and why? Was it a bit of both, perhaps? Were threats or tears involved? Or were you like Adam Sandler's character, having a hard time noticing or acknowledging your angry feelings?

Western culture has such a negative outlook of anger that we try very hard to suppress it. It's an uncomfortable experience for many of us, and we want

---

27. *Anger Management*, Peter Segal, director. Produced by Columbia Pictures, Revolution Studios, Happy Madison Productions. Released April 11, 2003.

it to be over as soon as possible. In many self-development or spiritual communities, those who are angry can be dismissed as having poor character or accused of being spiritually inept. There's a high value placed on peace, forgiveness, and compassion. Spiritual work is often focused on transcending and rising above our anger.

Not to play word games here, but how do you *rise above* something that's very nature is to rise? We do a lot of emotional gymnastics to move away from anger. Because of this, we can overlook the fact that anger is a cue from our internal self that something needs to change. When we either try to get rid of that anger or express it recklessly—without dealing with the underlying call for change—we create all kinds of *wahala* in our bodies, souls, and lives. (*Wahala* is a Nigerian slang word that means "chaos" or "trouble." It's my favorite word, and I've been dying to add it to this book.) When we learn to get comfortable with conflict, respond appropriately, our qi flows so that change in evolution and growth can happen.

Women in general, and Black women in particular, are demonized for getting angry. In a study on gendered racism in the workplace, researchers discovered that Black women who diverge from the image of the modern mammy, women who "uphold white-dominated structures, institutions or bosses at the expense of their personal lives," risk being perceived as the "Black Bitch" archetype.[28] Dr. Harriet Lerner elaborates on the challenge women face in her book, the *Dance of Anger*:

> The direct expression of anger, especially at men, makes us unladylike, unfeminine, unmaternal, sexually unattractive, or, more recently, "strident"…Our language condemns such women as "shrews," "witches," "bitches," "nags," "castrators". They are unloving and unlovable. They are devoid of femininity. Certainly, you do not wish to become one of them.[29]

28. Adia Harvey Wingfield, "The Modern Mammy and the Angry Black Man: African American Professionals' Experiences with Gendered Racism in the Workplace," *Race, Gender & Class* 14, no. 1/2 (2007): 196–212.

29. Harriet Goldhor Lerner, *The Dance of Anger: A Woman's Guide to Changing the Patterns of Intimate Relationships* (New York: HarperCollins, 2014), 2.

Harmful stereotypes become cultural norms that keep women from accessing the anger of the Wood element in a healthy way. In addition to associating anger and assertiveness with a lack of femininity, we are used to seeing images of women characters such as Jean Grey of X-Men fame and Vanya of *The Umbrella Academy*, whose anger is an uncontrollable, destructive force. And let's not forget my favorite mad mama from *Game of Thrones*, Daenerys Targaryen. (Spoiler alert: if you haven't yet finished watching the series, you may want to skip to the next section. There will definitely be some spoilers!) By looking closely at this modern myth, we see a symbolic representation of what happens when a woman accesses the potent force of the Wood element.

Let me begin by offering some context to the story. King's Landing is the name of the city where Daenerys's, a.k.a Dany's, royal enemies live. These are the folks who killed the adults, children, and babies of her entire family. She and her brother barely escaped and now live in exile on the other side of the world. At the end of the eagerly anticipated eighth season, Dany uses her dragons to set the capital city of King's Landing ablaze. Viewers watch this destruction through the eyes of the villagers, running desperately for their lives. We see innocent children and homes consumed by flames and turned into piles of ash and dust. Daenerys prophetically reclaims her throne as the dreaded "Queen of the Ashes." After more than ten years of watching Dany grow into her queendom, her uncontrollable anger and rage become her demise. If only she had listened to her wise counselor when he advised that she spare King's Landing (insert sarcastic eye roll).

What was painfully absent from the post-GOT finale buzz was a conversation about the fact that Dany accomplished exactly what she set out to do. In season one, when we meet her being pawned off as a sex slave for her brother's gain, we learn that her prophesied purpose in life is to avenge her family's ruin. When she is later sold as a wife to hottie Khal Drogo, they vow to cross the seas together to destroy King's Landing so that she can reclaim her rightful place on the Iron Throne. She eats a raw horse heart to ritualistically seal this destined deal. From their unlikely birth, she raises her baby dragons with the vision of one day burning King's Landing to the ground. In Wood element fashion, on her quest she conquers cities, frees slaves, and burns alive those who threaten justice or her leadership. When she hesitates, one of her fierce woman allies advises her to stop playing small and "be a dragon."

Dany wasn't mad with rage or blinded by emotions when she attacked King's Landing. True to the Wood element, she had a vision and executed her plan with unwavering, single-pointed focus. I mean sure, she was hurt when her enemies executed her closest friends. Who wouldn't be? But, she destroyed King's Landing as part of a sophisticated war strategy, and as a step toward her lifelong goal of sitting on the Iron Throne. As the general of her army, she gave the command and executed the plan.

I get fired up by this story (pun intended) because so often our culture a labels a woman as "hysterical" or "mad" when she displays strong emotions. When a so-called crazy woman is enraged, it is easy to dismiss her brilliance and her accomplishments. And that is exactly what happened to Dany. Instead of being remembered for the cities she freed and the lives she liberated, she goes down in history like her father, as the "Mad Queen." *Game of Thrones* ends with her assassination celebrated as a heroic act.

Rather than demonizing Dany, we can better understand the Wood element if we align her symbolic story with goddesses from the myths of ancient cultures. Like Dany, you don't want to get on the bad side of these divine feminine forces of destruction. There's Pele, the fiery volcano goddess of the Pacific Islander tradition. There's Oya, the warrior goddess of the African Diasporic spiritual pantheon, who serves as the inspiration for the X-Men character Storm. Kali, of the Hindu faith is known as the Destroyer. All of these goddesses can come to wreck shit, but they are also necessary forces of transformation. They are forces of nature that personify the fierce, eruptive power of the Wood element when divine justice must be served. Whenever I feel hesitant to express my anger or feel tempted to back down, I call to mind the quote by American author Charles Bukowski: "She's mad, but she's magic. There's no lie in her fire."[30]

Speaking of justice, do you know who else is not allowed to be angry in America? Black men. The image of the "threatening Black man" is very much embedded in the psyche of American culture, and the portrayal of Black men as lustful, brutal rapists has been used to justify lynchings, police brutality, and systemic oppression. Because of this, many Black men have learned to

30. "A Quote by Charles Bukowski," Goodreads, accessed October 18, 2021, https://www.goodreads.com/quotes/1014889-she-s-mad-but-she-s-magic-there-s-no-lie-in-her.

quiet and suppress their anger, so as not to become threatening to their peers. South African comedian and television host Trevor Noah explains:

> I grew up learning one thing: it's way easier to be an angry white man than an angry black man...White people—for the most part—have always had their anger heard. When white people complain, shit gets done, it gets changed. Black people have learned you need to find subtle ways to get your point across.[31]

His words resonate deeply with what I have witnessed in the men of my family and closest friends, many whom have developed sophisticated strategies to avoid making others uncomfortable in their presence. It's no wonder that facing discrimination and microaggressions has been linked to chronic muscular tension and pain,[32] a key diagnostic signature of the Wood element. When Black men are angry (and even when they aren't), they are perceived as a threat and the ultimate enemy. The pressure to face daily, relentless injustice and to *not* be able to get angry about it is the epitome of unfair. And the Wood element doesn't like it.

To date I've seen *Black Panther* about twelve times (and counting). The movie is based on a comic book that strongly resonates with the Wood element's impulse for revolution and self-determination. The cinematic masterpiece is rich with powerful archetypes—including the late Chadwick Boseman in an incredible performance in the title role, and my celebrity crush, Michael B. Jordan, as Erik Killmonger. Killmonger is a warrior who represents the best and worst of the Wood element. He wants justice at any cost. His vision is to arm the oppressed with Vibranium, and he devises a plan to send weapons to colonized people in major cities around the world. He aims to start a revolution that would usurp unjust power dynamics. I am still confused by why we collectively cheered when those weapons never left Wakanda! But our reaction to this modern myth further illustrates that there are huge, unconscious discrepancies in who is allowed access to the Wood element's call for anger, justice, and revolution.

---

31. Lanre Bakare, "Trevor Noah: 'It's Easier to Be an Angry White Man than an Angry Black Man,'" The *Guardian*, April 2, 2016.

32. Timothy T. Brown et al., "Discrimination Hurts: The Effect of Discrimination on the Development of Chronic Pain," *Social Science & Medicine* 204 (2018): 1–8.

Clearly, we have a lot of work to do to reconcile our collective relationship with anger. Despite its bad reputation, anger is good for us. Remember, the Wood element supports the fullest expression of our individual greatness. If we don't have the capacity to get angry when we are violated, it means our ability to individuate has been compromised. It's unhealthy. The purpose of anger is to preserve the integrity of the self. A healthy Wood element will respond (with minor irritation or full blown rage) to any of the following triggers that threaten our integrity. We know that anger is a signal for change when:

+ our freedom is obstructed;
+ an important emotional issue has not been addressed;
+ too many of our beliefs, values, desires, ambitions are being compromised;
+ we are doing or giving more beyond our capacity or more than is comfortable;
+ others are doing too much at the expense of our competence and growth;
+ our boundaries are being violated, or our "no" is not being heard; and
+ we are not being seen or validated.[33]

This list is not exhaustive, and certainly there may be other situations that trigger righteous indignation. But healthy anger is usually a response to one of the above. As you reflect on the last time you were angry, can you identify any of these triggers working behind the scene?

As we review this list of triggers, we get insight into to why racism, sexism, patriarchy, and other forms of systemic oppression are such triggers for anger and social unrest. That's the Wood element's job—it rises up to protect freedom and justice for all. If someone or something is blocking my freedom, the Wood element will support my absolute right to take a stand (soul lesson 2), express myself (soul lesson 3), and pursue my purpose (soul lesson 4). There's going to be some anger for sure, and that anger serves as a motive force. The Wood element teaches us how to work with our anger—not as something to

---

33. Lorie Dechar, Alchemical Healing Weekend Training, March 2017.

transcend or suppress—but as an energy to harness as we listen to its message for our growth and expansion.

Reflection Questions

How do you deal with your anger? Take a moment to reflect on the following questions in your journal:

+ Who or what makes you angry?
+ How do you typically express your anger?
+ How do you respond to anger in others?
+ Can you think of a time when your anger propelled you to make an important change?
+ How is anger regarded in your spiritual practice or religion?
+ What did you learn about anger from your family of origin? Are there any wounds that need to be addressed?

Flower Essences to Facilitate Healthy Relationship with Anger

The following flower essences help us to listen to our anger and use it as a tool for transformation and growth:

+ Dandelion to release the tension
+ Willow to dissolve resentment
+ Blue Elf Viola to speak from the heart

Dandelion: Release the Tension—Dandelion is a very popular and potent flower! It is one of those very first flowers to emerge in the spring here in New York. It's bright and bold and beautiful. And then it softens: dandelion's golden fashion statement transforms into a soft puff we can blow into the wind with a wish. In herbal circles, dandelion is pretty well known for its liver detoxification benefits, even more deeply aligning the plant with the Wood element. When considering its properties as a flower essence, we are considering how Dandelion's softening and cleansing qualities impact our psycho-emotional well-being.

Plants often grow natively in the environments where they have the most wisdom to share. In fact, getting to know the wildflowers of a particular area will hint at the soul qualities the humans who live there are wrestling with.

It's not a surprise that dandelion grows so wildly abundant in the city, because this flower addresses the embodied stress of the daily hustle and grind. When I see a dandelion on my morning walk, I envision a reassuring nod from Mother Nature saying, "I got you, girl!"

Dandelion flower essence is used to release emotional tension stored in the muscles. It is an ally for chronic embodied tension when the Wood element's desire to achieve makes us push ourselves too hard. While working with Dandelion, many of my patients begin to acknowledge the unaddressed stressors they've been holding in their bodies. Though what they've held is often anger and frustration, any negative emotion can cause stagnation in the free and easy flow of their lives. Physical symptoms of embodied stress include neck and shoulder tension, indigestion, irregular or painful menstrual cycles, and tension headaches. Dandelion gifts us with an awareness of what we are holding in our bodies instead of addressing in our lives.

Overwork becomes a way to avoid confronting these deeper emotions, and it adds more stress on top of them. Dandelion swoops in and whispers, "Settle down, calm down." We receive insight into how to create a release valve for the building pressure such as seeing a therapist, hitting the gym, journaling, or scheduling a biweekly massage. In fact, adding Dandelion flower essence to a few drops of olive oil makes for a very soothing massage or bath oil at the end of an emotionally tense day.

Just like the fluffy puffball that we can blow into the wind, Dandelion flower essence supports us in softening to our stress. While working with Dandelion, the initial response may be a sense of release and ease. With longer use, Dandelion supports an awareness of buried emotional treasures waiting to be released into the wind.

Willow: Release Resentment—Willow flower essence is indicated for bitterness, resentment, and unexpressed anger. This emotional holding pattern keeps us locked in the past, and creates stagnation for the Wood element that desires to push forward. Willow helps to break up and dissolve crystallized bitterness and resentment that creates stagnation in our emotional flow.

The *I Ching*, the divination text of ancient China, gives insight into how unresolved and suppressed anger affects our life. The eighteenth hexagram is called *ku*, or "decay." Its symbolic image is festering worms in a bowl.[34] Imagine a plate with food scraps that accidentally falls behind your couch—out of sight, out of mind. As the food scraps rot, stuff starts to grow. After a while it starts to stink, and you have to look all over to find out where the funk is coming from. Pretty gross, right?

Unresolved anger does the same thing. Something happened, and instead of dealing with it, we just stuffed it down or forgot about it. But it festers and spoils and gets more and more invasive until it smells bad enough for us to do something about it. By the time we find it, its unrecognizable. The eighteenth hexagram instructs us to "work on what has been spoiled." In other words, you gotta clean out the pot so that life can start flowing again. Willow flower essence helps us to get all the gunk out so that we can have a clean start.

Sometimes we are not conscious of the resentment that we are holding. This will manifest as a relationship wrought with tension and ongoing conflict that seems to come out of nowhere. You know those relationships where suddenly you are arguing about something really silly? You feel emotionally distant or easily agitated around this person. Sarcasm seeps into your conversations, conveying latent animosity. Or, we just don't know why we're tense and find it easier to avoid a person altogether than to deal with the discomfort. Willow will support us as we explore the underlying roots of our tension and aversion. It will awaken the awareness of why resentment is there in the first place, bringing to the surface unresolved conflicts or places where our Wood element felt violated. In some cases, we can see that the cause of our resentment has nothing to do with the other person, or we can receive deeper insight into the circumstances that were beyond anyone's control.

When we are consciously aware of resentment we are holding, we usually have an accompanying narrative that helps us to hold on to the hurt. We buy into the story we've created about how we've been wronged or violated. Even when this anger is justified, something in the natural flow of anger has gone awry. For whatever reason, the conflict was never resolved, and we're left carrying a big old bag of bad feelings. In these scenarios, Willow helps us acknowledge the moment when our own choices contributed to the conflict.

---

34. Richard Wilheim and Cary F. Baynes, *The I Ching or Book of Changes* (Princeton, NJ: Princeton University Press, 1967), 39.

This does not absolve the other party of their wrongdoing. However, we are not victims. Willow affirms our personal responsibility and agency, inviting us to choose a different path in the future. It also helps us see that in most cases, folks are not looking for our toes to stomp on! Rather, we gain the perspective that the transgressions that happen in relationships are an inevitable part of the human story, and are opportunities to grow. This self-awareness frees the Wood element to let go and move forward. There may even be space for compassion and forgiveness, or reestablishing a relationship that honors the integrity of all parties involved. Willow teaches us that moving forward is not mandatory but is always an option.

Blue Elf Viola: Speak from the Heart—Blue Elf Viola is a flower essence that supports honest communication when we are feeling upset or angry. It helps us find the right words to express the change that our Wood element is asking for. Blue Elf Viola is an ally for times when you don't want to avoid conflict but also don't want to walk into a disagreement with guns blazing. Instead, the goal is to clearly articulate the source of the upset, as well as what needs to be done to rectify it.

Anger is one emotion that easily disguises others. This flower essence supports emotional integrity, and helps us come to terms with anger that may be masked by fear or sadness. Blue Elf Viola is a good personal friend of mine. I used to be that person who, whenever I got angry, I would start crying. I would try to talk, and it would just all fall apart into a sniffling, snotty mess. I just could not articulate why I was angry. There was no growth because I wasn't saying what needed to be said. Ten years later, I was still mad. The other person never had to correct their violation because the attention was focused on the aforementioned snotty mess. So there was no healing. Gradually, with Blue Elf Viola's help, I have learned to connect to my heart while expressing my hurt.

This vibrant indigo flower essence opens our communication, especially in tense situations, and extra-especially in those situations where someone clearly needs to be checked, but you want to do it in a way that honors yourself *and* the relationship. It reminds us that the goal of confrontation is not to destroy the relationship or even to be right, but to evolve. When we are feeling congested, muddled, or unclear, Blue Elf Viola helps us to breathe into our hearts and to allow our hearts to speak. BlueEelf Viola is a flower essence that helps to condense the time gap between our feelings of anger and righteous indignation, and the expression of ourselves in a heart-centered way that preserves our integrity. You know that time gap, when the insight into what you "shoulda said" hits you a full three weeks after the conversation! Blue Elf Viola helps us express our heartfelt emotions while staying connected to love, especially when we're angry.

I also offer Blue Elf Viola to my revolutionary and activist colleagues, who share hard truths in their writing or public speaking. Even though they are not particularly angry, I have found that this essence supports them as they advocate for social change and world evolution. By staying connected to their heart, their personal experience and vulnerability rings triumphant in their words. Blue Elf Viola reminds us that when we speak our heart-centered truth, we wield tremendous political and spiritual power.

Embodied Practice: Utthita Trikonasana (Triangle Pose)

Affirmation: Anger is the energy of change.

In mathematics, the Greek symbol delta is an upward pointed triangle that stands for "change." To embody this symbol, begin by taking a wide step forward, forming a triangle with your legs. Extend your arms in a wide T. Hinge at the waist, drawing you lower arm to rest on your front foot by your calf or on a block as your upper arm reaches toward the sky.

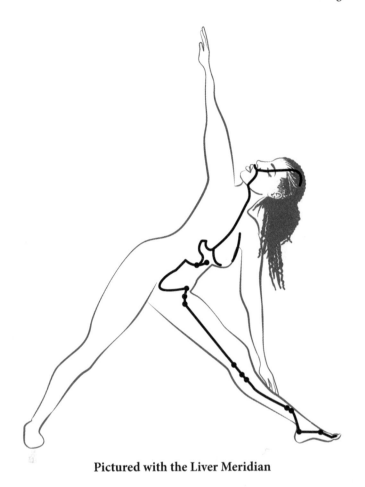

Pictured with the Liver Meridian

Call to mind a situation that is causing tension or conflict. Imagine the opposing perspectives as the base of a triangle. Envision those tension points moving toward resolution at the upper point of the triangle. Recite the affirmation: *Anger is the energy of change.*

Repeat on the opposite side.

Soul Lesson 2: Take a Stand

When I dare to be powerful—to use my strength in service of my vision,
then it becomes less and less important whether I am afraid.
—Audre Lorde

We can deepen our understanding of this soul lesson by looking at the symbolic language of Chinese Medicine. In pinyin, the character for anger is *nu*. Elisabeth Rochat de la Vallée, a linguist, sinologist, and scholar, explains that in the upper left portion of this character is a mark that symbolizes a woman along with a character for a hand. The mark at the bottom of the character is the symbol for "heart." (This is known as a radical, a character that broadly categorizes its word as belonging to a certain family. In this case, the heart radical tells us that this character symbolizes an emotion.) She describes this character as "the natural feeling of a woman under the hand of someone."[35] Rochat goes on to explain that in a dictionary of Chinese *hanzi* (characters), *nu* is transliterated as "a female slave under the hand of a master."[36] The character conveys one emotional complexity of the Wood element, the suppressed anger of a person who is being oppressed.

The character *nu* refers to powerlessness or rage that is as much an expression of the Wood element as is the yelling, screaming, fighting, and all the things we typically associate with anger. When the Wood element is in disharmony, we feel oppressed, silenced, or trapped in our job, our marriage, our home, or any number of situations where we've lost our sense of personal agency. The feelings of powerlessness or resignation can easily translate into a form of depression. I ask the Wood element to support my patients who have run out of ideas and solutions. They feel like they've tried everything and that change is impossible. They are unable to see a way out. Their hopelessness and resignation remind me of a wilted plant, no longer reaching for the sun.

When we feel hopeless, part of what we are saying is "I can't see or imagine how this situation could be any different." That sinking hopelessness is an expression of a Wood element that is unable to rise up to the level of imag-

---

35. Claude Larre, Elisabeth Rochat de la Vallée, and Caroline Root, *The Seven Emotions: Psychology and Health in Ancient China* (London: Monkey Press, 2014), 65.

36. Ibid.

ining a new perspective or possibility. The Wood element restores hope and our vision for the change that is possible. Its signatures include not just having agency but also having somewhere to direct that strength of spirit. When we see the little light at the end of the tunnel, we have something to move toward. That forward movement lifts and rises against the sinking feelings of hopelessness, and we are able to step onto a path forward.

The Wood element teaches us how to transmute resignation into power and agency. Its natural energy is to rise. As it does, we learn how to take a stand. The Wood element affirms our right to exist, our right to take up space, our right to freedom, and our right to ease.

The Wood element is the archetype of the Spiritual Warrior, the one who fights for justice, speaks truth, and takes a stand in and for the world. It supports activists and those who are fighting the good fight in the struggle for justice and liberation. We call on the Wood element whenever there is a personal or collective violation that requires boundaries, advocacy, protection, or redemption. If necessary, the Wood element will go to war to protect equity and freedom. The Wood element is activated by the five faces of oppression:[37]

1. Exploitation: The act of using people's labor or genius to produce profit while not compensating them fairly.
2. Marginalization: When a group of people are relegated or confined to a lower socioeconomic standing or to the edges of society. For example, marginalized communities have less or substandard access to health care, education, quality food, and opportunities to build wealth.
3. Powerlessness: When a group of people is dominated by the ruling class and has zero or limited access to exercise their personal agency.
4. Cultural Imperialism: Involves establishing the values and norms of a dominant culture as the standard by which all other cultures are evaluated. Examples include the imposition of Eurocentric beauty standards, or discrimination against "foreign" language accents or dialects.
5. Violence: When members of some group live with the knowledge that they must fear random, unprovoked attacks on their person or

---

37. Adaptation of works by Iris Marian Young.

property simply because of who they are and what they represent. One example of violence is the 4,743 lynchings in the United States by the Ku Klux Klan from 1882 to 1968. This number does not include thousands of undocumented lynchings. [38]

The Wood element helps us restore our self-respect and dignity when we feel afraid to speak our truth or stand in our power. That fear may be rooted in ancestral memory of being stolen, terrorized, or annihilated. Maybe the fear is more immediate: I'm going to lose my job if I ask for the time off I need. I'm afraid maybe my relationship will not work out if I'm honest about my discomfort. Perhaps maybe my fear is that if I report my supervisor's sexual advances, I will jeopardize my career.

I have worked with clients in various stages of recovery from various types of physical, emotional, or sexual assault. I have witnessed the enormous shock, terror, pain, shame, and vulnerability involved. I have seen how trauma can live in our bodies, manifesting as numbness, anxiety, shame, and illness years after the abuse. Unhealed trauma rips apart the fabric of families and communities for generations. The Wood element helps us to feel solidity of the earth beneath our feet as we push up and rise toward change. It offers perseverance and tenacity when our right to exist is threatened, disregarded, or violated.

The Wood element supports both the bully and bullied, and I can think of no bigger bully than white supremacy. In 2020 when the videos of George Floyd's murder went viral, I was paralyzed with anger, fear, and grief. I got suspiciously quiet in social media, as no post could do anything about my broken heart. I felt deep despair for the countless lives lost: Breonna Taylor, Trayvon Martin, Eric Garner, Tamir Rice. Of course all lives matter. But the fact that I live in world where we have to specify that "Black Lives Matter"... well, *that also matters.*

---

38. "Lynching: By State and Race, 1882–1968" *Famous American Trials: The Trial of Joseph Shipp, et al.*: http://law2.umkc.edu/faculty/PROJECTS/FTRIALS/shipp /lynchingsstate.html.

I feel the trees looking down us with concern, thinking, "Humans, you've got to do better" as injustices against humanity are happening every day in every corner of the world. In the face of political turmoil, the Wood element offers us spiritual resilience to stay on purpose. The Wood element supported me through my feelings of anger, righteous indignation, and hopelessness, and inspired a deep desire to be of greater service to my community. It helped me understand that my path is not disconnected from all of this madness, but intrinsically connected. In fact, my very first elemental flower essence was created in response to the increase in police brutality incidents in the summer of 2016. I distributed the essences at a local yoga studio in Brooklyn as a soul heart balm. The flower essences shared in this section were part of that original flower essence remedy.

The Wood element teaches us that our genuine, authentic life purpose is not separate from the injustice we see in the world. In fact, it's just the opposite—the injustice is a challenge, a call to arms, a pleading of the universe to take a stand in service of humanity.

And let's be real: this political climate is calling for us *all* to stand up.

A call to all activists: stand up—oppression is a pandemic. We need your strategizing, your organization, your education, and your fight.

A call to all healers: stand up—hearts are broken, souls feel lost and confused, and trauma is real.

A call to all spiritualists: stand up—and help us raise the vibration of this planet.

A call to all families: stand up—let's raise our children to be change agents. Their eyes are watching.

A call to all lovers: stand up—love hard cuz love heals. Let's be forces of humility, honesty, caring, patience, validation, and compassion for one another.

And especially—a call to all of us with privilege: spiritual privilege, academic privilege, economic privilege, racial privilege. Let's be real about the privileges we have and use them to make space for those who don't have access.

The Wood element comes to shake shit up. As I write this chapter while remembering George Floyd and tallying lynchings, I feel my Wood element rise with equal parts rage, defiance, and resolve. I breathe into the stirrings of

Oya, the African warrior goddess of transformation who brings the storms of change. The discomfort we feel when the Wood element calls us to take a stand can be difficult, scary, and full of uncertainty. But the discomfort is also a necessary reminder that something is awakening. It's a reminder that we are sprouting. It's a reminder that all the seeds of renewal we planted are ready to crack, push against gravity, and rise up to the sun.

Reflection Questions

What is calling for you to take a stand? Take a moment to reflect on the following questions in your journal:

- What causes matter most to you?
- What privilege do you have, and how do you use it?
- Where do you experience discrimination or systemic oppression?
- Where do you push back against authority or the status quo?
- Who or what supports your self-actualization and individuality? Who or what stands in the way?
- What are the ways you make yourself small so that others can be more comfortable?
- Are there circumstances where your right to exist has been threatened or violated? What healing or support do you need?

Flower Essences to Take a Stand

Call on these allies from the flower essence world to help you stand firmly in your truth:

- Mountain Pride to awaken the spiritual warrior
- Goldenrod to resist social pressure
- Sunflower to be your own sun

Mountain Pride: Spiritual Warrior—Mountain Pride is in the *Penstemon* botanical family, all of whose flower essences support our tenacity and perseverance. Mountain pride blossoms in the mountain crevices, an adverse environment with tough terrains and climates that do not necessarily support growth and beauty. Yet it asserts its vibrant, rich color, thriving unapologetically and unexpectedly. This is a metaphor for Mountain Pride's effect on our psyche.

Mountain Pride supports you as you take a stand for your convictions as a spiritual warrior or within your community, relationship, or family. It's an amazing remedy when you need to stay the course, but lack the courage or will to fight. On a personal level, it's a great remedy to have on hand for those "hard-to-have" discussions at work or at home. In my clinical practice, Mountain Pride is an especially helpful flower essence for activists, as it helps them stay connected to their passion for social change when they feel burned out or defeated.

Mountain Pride emboldens our response to conflict, whether large-scale social injustices, or smaller personal conflicts that are necessary to the evolution of any relationship. In a personal conflict, this is the yelling, screaming, and fighting that follows a personal slight. On a social level, this is the outpouring of letters, protests, and marches, the flurry of activities with the goal of letting it be known that "we are not happy here!" We use our social media feeds to express our solidarity and educate our peers. This response gives us a place to discharge pent-up rage, dissatisfaction, and even fear so that we don't implode. It builds solidarity, confirming that we are not alone or isolated in our pain. This community in and of itself has healing power. When used strategically, our united front can put pressure on local officials or businesses to change policies and practices. We deepen our commitment to the fight for justice.

By their very nature, intense emotions (and media coverage) are short-lived. As the intensity fades, so does our ability to uphold many of the promises made at the height of emotion. Mountain Pride flower essence helps us process our intense emotions while offering insight into how to align our personal purpose with the fight for justice. This awakened power is easily sustained by love—of ourselves, our family, our community, and the world. Mountain Pride teaches how to confront adversity in a way that can be sustained for the long haul, even after media coverage ends. The flower essence also helps us to hold on to our inner peace while engaging in necessary, righteous struggle.

Speaking of peace, Mountain Pride is also an excellent plant remedy for spiritual bypassing, a term first coined by transpersonal psychologist John Welwood in his book, *Toward a Psychology of Awakening*.[39] It is defined as "using spiritual ideas and practices to sidestep personal, emotional 'unfinished business,' to shore up a shaky sense of self, or to belittle basic needs, feelings, and developmental tasks."[40] On a personal level, spiritual bypassing can be an excuse to turn to spiritual practices such as meditation to avoid conflict, difficult emotions, or unresolved wounds. On a social level, spiritual bypassing causes us to withdraw from engaging in social justice movements by asserting that the universe or a higher power will "take care" of things. In both scenarios, doing nothing is a form of denial or avoidance.

To be clear, spiritual bypassing is very different from spiritual *processing*. Our prayers have power. In many African Orthodox Christian communities, if someone says they will pray for you, they mean business. They will get up every morning at six a.m. and implore the spiritual realm to relieve your suffering. Other spiritual traditions perform elaborate rituals, chants, or prayers that seriously shift the underlying energies of pain and conflict. I've seen real miracles happen as a result of spiritual intervention.

But when we say, "I'll pray for you" to change the topic of conversation and never give it another thought, that's spiritual bypassing. When we turn our back on the suffering of others, pretending their pain doesn't exist because "everything has a higher purpose"? That's also spiritual bypassing. Spiritual bypassing shows up when we are "too enlightened" to do the work on the ground, and it is an insidious force within holistic and spiritual wellness communities.

Let me give you an example illustrating how spiritual bypassing works. Imagine I am in line at a grocery store, and the person in front of me accidentally pushes her cart back into me so much that it is resting on my foot. The cart is heavy and it hurts:

Me: Ouch! That really hurts!

---

39. John Welwood, *Toward a Psychology of Awakening: Buddhism, Psychotherapy, and the Path of Personal and Spiritual Transformation* (Boulder, CO: Shambhala, 2002).

40. "Spiritual Bypass," Wikipedia: https://en.wikipedia.org/wiki/Spiritual_bypass.

Them: (not turning to notice the cart on my foot): That's so interesting! I was just reading a book about how pain is an illusion.

Me: (getting annoyed) I need you to move your cart off of my foot.

Them: We are all connected. It's not my cart, it's *our* cart. I don't understand why we can't all just get along.

Me: (pushing the cart forcefully to liberate my now bruised and possibly broken foot)

Them: You need to work on your anger. I refuse to engage with toxic people.

Mountain Pride checks spiritual bypassing by challenging us to align our daily actions with our spiritual ideals, and encourages us to actively engage in service of our human family. Our response to conflict and injustice is not a one-size-fits-all kind of thing. Every situation is unique. Mountain Pride helps us determine the appropriate course of action for the situation. Is it being quiet and still, or is it fighting the fight? Is it being an ally and supporting those who have a clear vision and strategy or taking the lead? With Mountain Pride, we get clarity about the correct role to play. It helps us initiate purposeful, sustainable actions that connect our purpose to long-term change. Mountain Pride gives us insight into how exactly to lend our unique gifts, talent, brilliance, resources, and privilege to the struggle for justice.

Goldenrod and Sunflower: Push against Gravity—The Wood element gives us the potency, power, vision, clarity, energy, and momentum to stand in our truth and to defy gravity, even if we're doing it alone. Sunflower and Goldenrod are two flowers that help us activate that aspect of the Wood element. Both are tall, vertical flowers that decisively reach for the sun. In addition, their golden color resonates with the solar plexus, the energy center that is the seat of our self-actualization and personal power.

What now seems like a million years ago, the *Wizard of Oz* movie would air every year on Thanksgiving. It seems impossible that this movie, one of the first to broadcast in color, is approaching a hundred years old! In the 1950s and '60s, the film deeply reinforced the mainstream values of America. It tells the story of Dorothy, a young farm girl whose house is swept up by a tornado, and lands in a mystical land. Her house lands on and kills the Wicked Witch of the East, which evokes celebration from the Munchkins who lived under her evil rule. In her quest, Dorothy must evade the Wicked Witch of the

West, and along the way she gains support from the magical, beautiful Glinda the Good Witch. Doe-eyed Dorothy Gale, played by Judy Garland, learns valuable lessons about friendship, purity, and innocence. The movie reinforced the popular belief at the time: there's no place like home.

As our society evolves, cultural myths get a reboot. In 1978, the *Wizard of Oz* was reintroduced as *The Wiz*, a musical with an all-Black cast and soundtrack featuring Diana Ross, Michael Jackson, and Richard Pryor. It has been a cult-classic in the Black community for decades. Every summer the movie is played in Fulton Park in the historic Bedford-Stuyvesant, to the joy of the neighborhood kids (or terror … Evilline is legit scary). The movie got another reboot in the 2015 presentation of *The Wiz Live!*, staring hip-hop icons Common and Queen Latifah.

In 1995, author Gregory Mcguire created the backstory of the original *Wizard of Oz* with his novel, *Wicked: The Life and Times of the Wicked Witch of the West. Wicked* went on to become one of Broadway's most popular and critically acclaimed musicals. Right off the bat, *Wicked* beautifully illustrates signatures of the Wood element. First, the protagonist, Elphaba, is *green*, and she is discriminated against because of the color of her skin. And we know she is *angry*. After all, based on the original movie, we know that Dorothy just killed her sister and—with Glinda's support—takes the ruby red slippers off of her dead body. I mean, who murders someone and then steals their clothes? Talk about privilege! As the story unfolds, we get to question the status quo and our assumptions. Why is the witch wicked? Has she always been this way?

We eventually learn that Glinda the Good Witch and Elphaba went to high school together. When Elphaba walks into a room, people flinch; her very existence is an atrocity. Glinda, on the other hand, is popular. Her blonde hair, blue eyes, and wealthy background give her a leg up in the exclusive school. She's like a living Barbie doll—she has the hair, the body, and the flirtatious giggle that make her the golden girl. Glinda starts off as the ultimate mean girl and leads the charge teasing Elphaba because of her green skin, social awkwardness, and studious nature. Eventually, as forced roommates, the two become unlikely friends.

Just like in the original movie, we learn that the Wizard has no real power. Not only is he a fraud, he's also responsible for caging and silencing the mystical animals of Oz. Guess who figures out the diabolical shenanigans of the Wizard? And guess who really *does* have magic? Elphaba. When she decides to take a stand for the animals of Oz and speak truth to power, she is labeled as undeniably wicked. Elphaba must be demonized, because her truth could dismantle the whole fabric of Oz. Glinda, who is willing to keep the secrets of the janky wizard, gets put on a pedestal as the "Good Witch" we meet in the 1939 movie, traveling around in a bubble with sprinkles of magic. The song "Defying Gravity" marks the pivotal moment when Elphaba embodies the Wood element.

Both Goldenrod and Sunflower flower essences help us to embody the qualities Elphaba needs to become self-realized. She decides that she'd rather fly solo than be complicit and silent in the face of injustice. She bets on her own magic and power, and levitates up on out of Oz on her infamous broom.

Goldenrod: Resist Social Pressure—Goldenrod supports our ability to stand firmly in our personal truth in spite of influences from our social environment. With Goldenrod, we feel empowered to not waver against popular opinion. This flower essence is great support for kids experiencing peer pressure, as it is helps them center in their own understanding of right and wrong. We all experience the pressure to go with the flow, even when that flow runs against our personal current. As social beings, we are constantly under the influence of family, coworkers, media, friends, lovers—the list is endless. Goldenrod helps us identify those influences and make solid decisions that support our best interests. When working with Goldenrod, we are supported to say, "I can make a decision that's right for me. Even if it goes against the grain. Even if others think that I am wrong, or disagree. I can stand in what is true for me."

Without the ability to follow her own inner compass, Elphaba would have listened to a society that told her she was ugly and powerless. She would have believed that there was nothing she could do to fight against the injustices she witnessed. She also would have fallen in line with the foolishness of the powers that be without ever realizing her potential. Thank goodness Elphaba had the courage and the insight to resist outside influence and chart her own course. Goldenrod offers us the same gift.

Sunflower: Be Your Own Sun—Sunflower is another flower essence that helps us defy gravity. It is the flower essence that awakens the "I am-ness" of our being and a key flower essence to support self-actualization as we walk our destined path. Sunflower calls to us when we feel plagued with self-doubt and need a confidence boost. The flower supports the shining of our inner radiance, just like the glorious yellow flowers of this sunny plant.

When we work with Sunflower, we validate ourselves from within, instead of looking to others for approval. If Elphaba waited for others to give her permission to fly, she may have never achieved her greatness. When we see that light within ourselves, we have to nurture it. Sunflower also keeps us from being self-effacing. Sunflower brings our awareness to the many subtle ways we apologize for our existence. Have you ever said "sorry!" when someone bumped into you, even though it was clearly their fault? Do you brush off or discredit compliments when they are offered? Do you begin sentences with the phrase "I was just…," offering a disclaimer for what you are about to say, even before you say it? Do you talk fast so that others do not have to wait for you to complete your thoughts?

The sun does not apologize for shining. Sunflower helps us to tap into the radiance of our inner sun. We affirm "I am going after what is mine. I deserve it, and I am worthy." Sunflower reminds us that merely surviving isn't enough—we were born to thrive!

Embodied Practice: Virabhadrasana II (Warrior 2 Pose)

Affirmation: I stand in my power

Begin by facing the side wall of your space with your feet three to four feet apart. Turn your right foot ninety degrees, toes toward the front of your mat, so that your heel is perpendicular to your left foot. Slowly come into a steady lunge by bending your right knee until it is directly over your right ankle. Extend both arms out to the side, lifting and expanding through your chest. Gaze out over the tips of your right fingers. Press the outer edge of your left foot into the ground to engage the Wood element meridians in your legs.

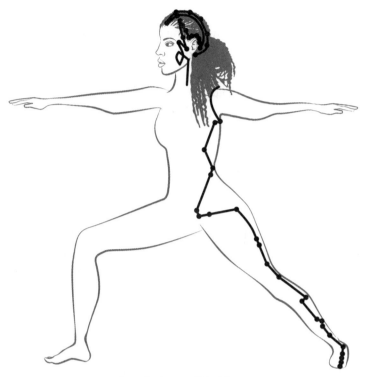

Pictured with the Gallbladder Meridian

Imagine that you are a spiritual warrior fighting for peace. Repeat the affirmation: *I stand in my power.*

Complete on the opposite side.

Soul Lesson 3: Express Yourself

Darling, you feel heavy because you are too full of truth. Open your mouth more. Let the truth exist somewhere other than inside your body.
—*Della Hicks-Wilson*

The Wood element teaches us how to express ourselves and speak our truth. This expression includes writing, public speaking, creative works, and any public performance. The Wood element also supports honest and authentic communication in our most intimate and personal spaces.

The teenage years awaken the Wood element's drive for self-discovery and self-definition. When I was in high school, I remember how desperately

I wanted to be seen, valued, and respected on my own terms. My brother, a superhuman scholar athlete who graduated as class valedictorian, was only two years ahead of me. I made it my mission to make a name for myself, lest I run the risk of being known as "Justin's little sister" for the rest of my life.

By luck or divine design, I landed a crew of friends who equally valued creative self-expression, originality, and authenticity. Once a month, sister-girlfriend, Amby-Am, would send out a call declaring the next day as a "Play Yo Self Day." These were days to completely abandon fashion rules and sensibilities with obnoxious patterns and colors. We would dress up in the most unconventional clothes we could find. A Burger King crown accessorized a gingham checkered apron-dress worn with black-and-white striped stockings. A lime green zoot suit joined forces with a neon orange polo shirt and polka-dot rubber rain boots. Anything that looked ridiculous was fair game. We closed out the year with a carefully choreographed performance of Salt 'N Pepa's "Expression" in the school talent show, a celebration of the wisdom conveyed through the song: you can only be yourself. The Wood element teaches us how to be authentic and creative. It supports us as we express ourselves through words, art, dance and the many ways we make our voices heard.

The pathways of the meridians clue us in to why the Wood element supports healthy self-expression. An internal branch of the Liver meridian traverses directly over the throat chakra. Like the Wood element, this chakra supports our ability to speak with clarity, and to express ourselves creatively. The throat chakra is related to any kind of creative expression. Chakra expert Anodea Judith speaks of the chakra as "the center of dynamic creativity, of synthesizing old ideas into something new. Its attributes include listening, speaking, writing chanting, telepathy, and any of the arts—especially those related to sound and language."[41]

When this vital energy center needs more flow, we often experience a sore or scratchy throat. One sure sign that the Wood element needs our attention is the sensation of what's known as Plum Pit Qi, which is described as a sensation of something being stuck in the throat. In my clinical practice, I've noticed that when a client is talking about something difficult, uncomfortable,

---

41. Anodea Judith and Lion Goodman, *Creating on Purpose: the Spiritual Technology of Manifesting through the Chakras* (Louisville, CO: Sounds True, 2012), 236.

or unresolved, they will instinctively bring their hand near their throat for support. This alignment of the throat chakra and the Liver meridian reminds us that our voice, our creativity, and the way we express ourselves are intimately connected to our agency and personal power.

There is a verse in the Bible that symbolizes the power of the spoken word as a creative force:

In the beginning, God created the heaven and the earth.

And the earth was without form, and void; and darkness was upon the face of the deep. And the Spirit of God moved upon the face of the waters.

And God said, Let there be light: and there was light.[42]

I have always been inspired the last bit of this verse in which God said, "Let there be light!" This closely resembles the ancient understanding that the sound is a vibration that becomes the manifested world. Our voice is often the gateway between what we think and what we manifest. In the manifestation process, conversation catalyzes.[43] Communication is an important step in moving a vision from mere imaginative fantasy into an actionable plan. Have you ever heard the folk superstition about not speaking something if you don't want it to be true? Whether we write it down in a journal or talk to a friend, the vibration of our words gives form and substance to our ideas.

Self-expression is also an important aspect of the healing process. In my practice, I pay close attention to my patient's willingness to speak openly about their experience. When they begin to share organically, I know healing is happening. The pain and trauma that remain unspeakable wreaks havoc on the psyche from the shadows. Their self-expression demonstrates that they feel safe enough to risk exposure, and to begin to control the narrative of the experience.

We can turn to the Wood element when we find it difficult to express ourselves or need extra support communicating with authenticity. If you're a writer, speaker, lawyer, student, teacher, or anyone who lives in a world that depends on clear communication, the Wood element helps you to use language masterfully. If, on the other side the spectrum, you tend to bite your tongue, the Wood element supports healthy expression and communication. If you tend to talk out

---

42. King James Bible, Genesis: 1–3

43. Anodea and Goodman, *Creating on Purpose*, 101.

the side of your neck and cause chaos with the things you say, working with the Wood element can help you adopt a healthier communication style.

Finally, the Wood element also invites us to use our voices as tools for personal and collective evolution. Not only do our words matter, there are also times when silence is violence. Harm persists when we don't speak up for ourselves and others. The silent treatment in intimate relationships can cause just as much emotional damage as verbal abuse. The Wood element challenges us to use our words in ways that matter—to heal, rather than to harm. There are times when it is difficult to know when to speak and when to be silent. A balanced Wood element helps us navigate these difficult conversations, written or spoken.

Reflection Questions

Are you ready to express yourself? Take a moment to reflect on the following questions in your journal:

+ How do you like to express yourself?
+ What are your creative outlets?
+ In which relationships are you able to express yourself easily?
+ In what circumstances do you bite your tongue?
+ How do you use your voice to advocate for others?
+ How do you communicate your boundaries? Is your strategy effective?

Flower Essences for Self-Expression

The following flower essences support our ability to express ourselves with confidence and creativity:

+ Trumpet Vine to turn up our volume
+ Calendula to soften our communication
+ Centaury to help us just say no

Trumpet Vine: Turn Up the Volume—Trumpet Vine looks like a little megaphone; as we would expect, it helps amplify our voice so that we can be heard. It's a great remedy for singers and actors who need to project their voices and have a strong presence. Trumpet Vine can raise the physical volume of a person's voice. I had one patient who I had to lean toward to hear what they were saying. After a few weeks working with Trumpet Vine, their voice was loud and clear. I no longer had to strain to listen to them, and they reported feeling more respected in their personal relationships.

However, Trumpet Vine does so much more than amplify our volume. It energizes our voices with qualities of the Wood element—assertiveness, clarity, and vitality. Classically, the Wood element is described as a shouting voice, but this often has nothing to do with being loud. A classical "Wood voice" is clear, direct, to the point, and knows where it's directed. Sometimes you almost want to duck out of the way! A voice without the Wood element's assertiveness is diagnosed as "Lack of Shout." The person may sound indecisive, wishy-washy, and timid. As a result, they are frequently not taken seriously and their boundaries are not respected. Trumpet Vine brings a vital, unapologetic quality to our self-expression.

Trumpet Vine gives us a voice that makes others sit up and listen. I often use Trumpet Vine with parents who are struggle with their rambunctuous children. Kids rely less on words, and more on energy for direction. They know, in spite of your threats to take away their toys or yelling and screaming, that you really ain't about that life. They are masterful at reading how serious we are, how much fight we have left in us, and they will manipulate the hell out of it. With Trumpet Vine, parents change the way they speak and, as my grandmother used to say, "put some bass in that voice." Children respond accordingly and know intuitively that the game is over.

In all relationships, Trumpet Vine helps us express our boundaries such that they are nonnegotiable. I use Trumpet Vine for clients who complain about not being taken seriously or being frequently interrupted in meetings. Trumpet Vine also supports my clients who find themselves having to constantly renegotiate their boundaries because they were not heard or respected the first time around. For writers, speakers, and performers, Trumpet Vine emboldens the written and spoken word with the vital, undeniable force of the Wood element. In all cases, Trumpet Vine helps our voices to be clear, direct, purposeful, and vibrant enough to inspire change.

Calendula: Soften the Edges—As a topical herbal remedy, calendula is often used for diaper rashes and sunburn. It cools the heat and softens, just like the calendula flower essence does for our communication. Calendula is a very useful flower for someone who is abrupt, brash, or caustic in their language. This person may also be argumentative or combative, or tends to rub other people the wrong way. Calendula helps to soften the edges of this type of communication, opening receptivity and grace in personal expression.

The person who needs Calendula has a quality in their voice that can be described as hostile, abrasive, demeaning, or condescending. They can't see that their words or tone is offensive, and are often confused by the constant miscommunication or conflicts they experience. Instead, they complain that others take what they say the wrong way. When we need Calendula, we end up in arguments and can't quite figure out how we got there. Like cream on a sunburn, Calendula flower essence softens the edges of that person's voice to cool the conflict.

Our capacity to listen and hear from the heart and our capacity to speak from the heart are interconnected. Calendula helps to soften our ears so that we can hear through the heart. This means we are receptive to the pure intention behind someone's words, no matter how those words come out. It's a great remedy when two people constantly argue but can't really hear what each other is saying.

Speaking of breakdowns in communication, let's talk about our favorite Wood element folks—teenagers! For adolescents, Calendula helps to soften the defensiveness that perhaps we all have when we're trying to assert ourselves. Teenagers are almost always primed for an attack, ready and waiting for people in authority to tell them "no." They've already got their defense locked and loaded, which creates an emotional holding pattern of tension, conflict, and struggle. Calendula whispers soothingly, "no one is trying to harm you or block your greatness." This helps them to be more receptive to their parents, teachers, mentors, and guides. It's not a cure for the necessary individuation teenagers need, but it does soften the way.

In all relationships, Calendula helps us drop our defenses, speak with kindness, and listen with a receptive heart. This is a particularly useful essence for conflict in interpersonal relationships you value and want to preserve. Let's be real: deep down, you know this person isn't a *total* idiot. Otherwise you wouldn't have married them/given birth to them/partnered with them, etc. There's some apparent love there, even though what and how they are communicating at the time is completely ridiculous (from your perspective). Calendula creates a bridge from heart to heart, so that there can be softness and receptivity in our communication.

Centaury: Just Say No—When my daughter was nine months old, I overheard her practicing how to say no in her crib. "NO!" she exclaimed with fierce authority. "Nooooooo?" she inquired, drawing out the syllable as if asking a question. "No…no…no," she admonished, mimicking my disciplinary style. She went on for about two minutes, experimenting with the word *no* in different tones. I kid you not, she was Nine. Months. Old. I couldn't believe it. Not only was "no" her first word, but she was already practicing how to say it. This young, powerful daughter of mine was born with her assertive Wood element intact. When I watch her navigate the world, I know the future is in good hands.

Like my daughter in her crib, Centaury flower essence helps us to learn many ways to say no. It teaches us the power of our "no," whether we express it with kindness or with unapologetic force. This flower essence could have easily been listed in the Earth element. As you will learn in a few chapters, the Earth and Wood elements represent a polarity within our psyche. I don't regard Earth and Wood as opposite ends of a spectrum. Instead, I envision the glyph used in astrology to represent the Sun: a circle with a dot in the center. The outer circle in this symbol represents the Earth element, and the dot as the networks of families and communities in which we are an interconnected is the Wood element. Like the sun itself, this dot symbolizes our individual ego, and the unique expression of ourselves. Centaury flower essence helps us to orient ourselves to that dot. From this central position, we learn how to set clear boundaries and to prioritize our own needs.

Like the centaur, the mythical half-human half-horse, Centaury addresses our core solar plexus consciousness and the confidence to assert necessary boundaries. A person who needs Centaury may feel like a doormat or be resentful or weary from always being considered last. They often feel unappreciated, yet incapable of putting their foot down. Centaury teaches us how to say no to others so that we can say "YES!" to ourselves.

Embodied Practice: Matsyasana (Fish pose)

Affirmation: My expression is a creative force.

Lie on your back with your legs extended flat in front of you. Place your hands palms down underneath your hips, propping yourself on your elbows as you lift your chest toward the sky. Tilt your head back to rest on the floor or a block, offering a gentle stretch in your throat chakra.

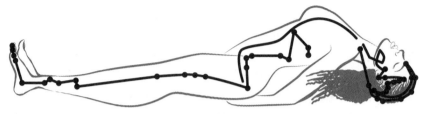

Pictured with the Gallbladder Meridian

Envision your words cascading from your heart, through your throat and entering the world through your voice. Use a deep hum, sensing the vibration of sound as it reverberates through your body. Repeat the affirmation: *My expression is a creative force.*

Soul Lesson 4: Your Purpose Has Power

"We're here to put a dent in the universe.
Otherwise why else even be here?"
—Steve Jobs

Do you, boo. YOLO (You Only Live Once). Live your best life. All of these are phrases we use when we are living into the Wood element. Think about that first day in early spring, when you sense the season changing. There is an expansive feeling that any- and everything is possible. The budding trees and singing birds fill us with hope, and awaken a sense of abundance and ease. We call on the Wood element to support us when we're ready to experience the best life has to offer as an innovator, visionary, entrepreneur, or creative. The Wood element supports us as we discover our true, authentic purpose.

Let's revisit the character *nu* from a few soul lessons ago. You may remember that this character depicts anger, the emotion associated with the Wood element. A second translation of the same character is "the effort to raise something up from the earth's gravity."[44]

In the mythology of Chinese Medicine, the great fish of the ocean of the northern abyss transforms into a majestic bird. The character *nu* describes the

---

44. Larre, Rochat de la Vallée, Root, *Seven Emotions*, 64.

energy required for the fish to swim, rise up, and transform into the flying bird. Can you imagine that little fish right before it takes that leap? It's looking at the sky and thinking, "This swimming thing is cool, but I'm actually meant to fly." That's how we feel when the Wood element is pushing us into our destined greatness. The rising of Wood element Qi is the natural expression of us becoming greater and greater beings.

My office has about a bazillion plants. Each of them, in their own way, is looking for light. Some of the plants require a lot of sun, while others are happy in the shade. Some of the plants reach and stretch around something blocking it—a fence, another tree, bad placement in a corner. In a similar way, Wood gifts us with the tenacity and determination to reach our goals. The Wood element is often symbolized by a bamboo plant, a metaphor for our ability to move with the wind and bend without breaking, to be flexible as we navigate the path to our purpose.

In the Water element, we gain insight into the destiny we are born into, which is outside our control. We can consider the Water element soil we are planted in. Our families, the home or city we were raised in, our skin color, our genetics—there's not much we can do to change any of those things. The Wood element emerges out of Water with a defiant "No matter what kind soil I've been planted in, I'm gonna thrive." Born into racism? Born into poverty? Born into poor health? The Wood element takes a defiant stance with a resounding, "I will rise." I read the entire poem "Still I Rise" by Maya Angelou as a tribute to the magnificence of the Wood element. The Wood element makes us adaptable to our conditions, yet determined to rise in spite of them. The people, institutions, and circumstances that stand in the way of our greatness are also checked by a healthy dose of the Wood element.

We are all familiar with the survival instinct. Our survival instinct doesn't just keep us alive, it also makes us hardwired to do whatever we have to do to feel safe and secure. The survival instinct will drive a starving person to eat dirt and drink their own urine. The survival instinct will also drive us to lie, cheat, and steal if we have to. It's a powerful force. There is an equally powerful and strong instinct within us to live our best life, called the entelechy. In the *Alchemy of Inner Work*, Lorie Dechar and Benjamin Fox (two of my favorite alchemical wizards) describe this instinct:

The word [entelechy] is made up of two parts: the first part, *en*, means "to have," the second *telos*, means "completion." Entelechy suggests that my beginning also contains my end. Its means that life had an innate, inborn purpose and direction. From the perspective of entelechy, spirit infuses for and matter with divine intention. Consciousness is going somewhere, and you too have a destiny, and implicit wholeness and completion already in you at the moment of your birth."[45]

It blows my mind to know that we are instinctively driven to realize our gifts and talents, and to become who we are meant to be.

Tao is a term that describes the universal way, the way of nature, and universal law. It is the inherent oneness of the entire universe of which humans are but a small part. I envision the Tao as a large interconnected spiderweb of divine design. This web consists of threads that reflect every single aspect of creation. The threads are intricately woven in such a way that not one thread can be removed without unraveling the entire fabric of the universe. Each of us is a thread in this web, and our unique thread is our personal Tao. Our spirit, purpose, and destiny are interconnected with the soul of the entire cosmos.

When we honor our entelechy, driving us to the fulfillment of our personal tao, we experience prosperity and abundance. This is because the universe wants us to be successful as we maintain our thread in the cosmic web. Our personal Tao plays an important role in universal tao. We may not be able to perceive the magnitude of universal Tao (it's above our pay grade as mere mortals). Yet when we follow our personal Tao, we get signs—in the form of resources, creativity, ideas, vision, inspiration, and blessings—to keep going. It's all connected in the web of life. Trust me when I tell you that the universe has your back. The Wood element is responsible for this self-actualization.

Abundance comes from being grounded and clear in our purpose, and able to use the gifts we are given to their fullest expression. It's a synergistic relationship: what we do for the world, the world does for us. We can release the struggle, the fear, and the fight, and allow the Tao to have her way with us. And when we don't? Well, the Wood element starts speaking loudly in the form of depression, irritability, and hopelessness as our deferred dreams dry

---

45. Dechar and Fox, *Alchemy of Inner Work*, 48.

up like raisins in the sun.[46] We are plagued with self-doubt, confusion, or anxiety. Sometimes, we experience blocks or obstructions, which were set in our path to guide us back to our destiny. As my therapist eloquently reminds me, "spirit is either preparing you … or protecting you."[47]

The Wood element helps us gain insight into our personal thread in the interconnected web of the universal Tao. It helps us intuit and follow our personal Tao and clarifies our values, our vision, and our place in the world as we pursue our purpose.

Reflection Questions

Are you living on purpose? Take a moment to reflect on the following questions in your journal:

+ What is your passion project?
+ How do you use your gifts and talents?
+ If money and time were of no concern, how would you spend your days?
+ What lights you up?
+ When do you feel most abundant?
+ What limiting beliefs do you have about doing the work you truly love?

Flower Essences to Align with Our Purpose

The following essences help connect us to our purpose and walk our destined path:

+ Wild Oat for passionate purpose
+ Lady Slipper to stand in inner authority
+ Scleranthus for clear decision-making
+ Blackberry to take decisive action

Wild Oat: Passionate Purpose—The Wood element offers clarity on how we can use our unique talents and gifts to lead a meaningful, purposeful life. The universe is always advocating for us to be our greatest self, and constantly opens doors of opportunity for us. Wild Oat helps us walk through those open doors and pay attention to the signs that we are on the right path.

---

46. Langston Hughes, "'Harlem,'" in *The Collected Works of Langston Hughes* (Columbia, MO: University of Missouri Press, 2002).

47. Dr. Maat Lewis, conversation with the author, August 2021.

When using Wild Oat, we notice benevolent coincidences and synchronicities that are like the bread crumbs on the path to our goals. If we trust and follow the bread crumbs, we find ourselves being in the right place, at the right time, with the right people, saying the right thing! In short, we end up exactly where we're supposed to be.

Wild Oat is a great ally when we are soul-searching. It was one of the most popular essences in my clinical practice when the COVID pandemic took its economic toll. Entire industries closed, work spaces shifted, and many of us began to question in earnest what we wanted to do "when we grew up." In a Wild Oat state, we dibble and dabble in various hobbies, jobs, careers, and projects, but are not fulfilled. Our heart just isn't in it. Wild Oat helps us discover the places where we feel truly alive and on purpose. The essence might spark the determination to make a career change. It can also inspire new creative projects, meaningful volunteer work, or any number of ways for us to lend our gifts to the world. When we work with Wild Oat, we discover new ways to find meaning and purpose, as well as work that lights up our soul. One of my clients working with Wild Oat discovered her love for painting. This did not mean she was destined to become a professional painter; instead, the creative space allowed her to gain perspective, clarity, and vision. Painting opened her creativity, which she then applied to her lifework in the nonprofit sector.

While working with Wild Oat, a friend introduced me to the Japanese concept of *ikigai*, translated as "purpose" or "reason for being." In *Ikigai: The Japanese Secret to a Long and Happy Life*, authors Héctor García and Francesc Miralles explain the Japanese characters in the phrase *ikigai* combine ones that mean "life," "to be worthwhile," "taking initiative as a leader," and "beautiful" or "elegant."[48] Altogether, *ikigai* is understood as the path we take to lead a worthwhile and beautiful life. The Wood element in general and Wild Oat flower essence specifically supports us in this endeavor. An *ikigai* consists of a Venn diagram of overlapping spheres of influence that ask four questions:

+ What do you love?
+ What does the world need?
+ What are you good at?
+ What can you be paid for?

---

48. Héctor García, Francesc Miralles, and Heather Cleary, *Ikigai: The Japanese Secret to a Long and Happy Life* (New York: Penguin Books, 2017), 11–12.

Our ikigai is at the intersection of our passion, our mission, our vocation, and our profession. Wild Oat facilitates an embodied exploration of our *ikigai*, and reminds us that we are not defined by how much money we make or what we do for a living. Rather, it inspires us to structure our lives such that we can fulfill our purpose in the interconnected web of the universe.

Lady's Slipper: Inner Authority—While Wild Oat offers insight into our purpose, Lady's Slipper awakens the inner authority to walk our path. Lady's Slipper helps us to root our daily actions to our larger purpose. We reclaim the power and the confidence to assert: "I've got the goods to do what I'm here to do."

Because of patriarchy and racism, some of us need some extra support to recognize our authority. Think about it. Every single practice discussed in the book comes from Brown cultures: yoga originated in India, mindfulness meditation descends from an East Asian Buddhist lineage, Chinese Medicine was preserved through Taoist alchemists in China, and archetypal self-awareness is rooted in traditional African spiritual systems. Yet many of the current mainstream voices on these matters are white men, followed by white women.

I love Sebene Selassie's *You Belong: A Call to Connection.*[49] Rooted in the Black and immigrant experience, Sebene introduces Buddhist meditation as an art that is embodied, political, relational, and transformative. It has changed my experience of meditation. *You Belong* does something that, unfortunately, is still considered a radical idea: it presents a Black woman as a voice of wisdom and authority in the wellness field to non-Black audiences.

I met Sebene a bazillion years ago when we worked together at a small social justice nonprofit organization. We often joke about how we've both ended up in the healing arts and the paths we took that led to our shared conclusion that what the world really needs right now is a soul makeover. Sebene has offered so much encouragement in my book writing journey. I shopped this book for over two years before finding an agent and then another before finding a publisher. That kind of rejection can do a number on your self-esteem. Sebene encouraged me to keep going and recalled that the word "author" is the root of "authority." She reminded me of the two decades of inner work, ten years of clinical practice, multiple graduate degrees, and the personal commitment that qualifies me as authority in my field. And like Lady's Slipper flower essence, she helped me break through the insecurity,

---

49. Sebene Selassie, *You Belong: A Call for Connection* (New York: HarperOne, 2021).

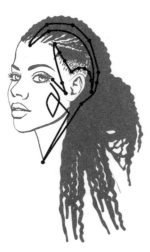

4.3 Close-up of Gallbladder Meridian

self-doubt, and nervous exhaustion that arise when we are unable to fully embody the steps on our destined path.

Asé (pronounced ah-SHAY) is a West African philosophical concept that refers to the spiritual power to make something happen. It's like the stamp of approval from the gods that gives us the spiritual authority to do something because it is part of our destiny. When we say *Asé!* at the end of a statement, it's the equivalent of saying, "so be it," "it is so," or "it's a done deal!" It's similar in essence to the Arabic word *maktub*, which means "it was written," and the Southern colloquial expression, "from your lips to His ears." When something has the spiritual *Asé*, it can undoubtedly manifest in the physical world.

When we have the *Asé* to do something, we don't need permission or validation from others. Lady's Slipper helps us connect to the inner knowing of our destiny, so that we can be unwavering and committed as we walk our path on Earth. The flower essence helps us to cultivate the healthy self-righteousness of the Wood element. Instead of relying on others to approve us, we tap into our inner spiritual authority and agency. We release the anxiety of wondering what will happen, and trust that things will unfold as they should. We know that what's for us is *for us*. We don't have to send out an army of defenses and back-up plans on our life path. Instead, the juicy, delightful steps into our inner authority allow us to dance our destined path with grace, joy, and ease.

Scleranthus: Clear Decision-Making—The Gallbladder in Chinese Medicine takes decisive actions and makes clear choices to move us along our destined path. The meridian zigzags across the head and then continues to zigzag down our body. It's as though the meridian can't make up its mind about which path to take! [**Figure 4.3**] When this energetic channel is imbalanced, we experience aches and pains that alternate from one side to another or that come and go. In our psyche, this manifests as indecision or flakiness.

The Scleranthus flower essence facilitates clear, decisive decision-making when we are faced with two comparable options. Whenever this flower pops up in my clinical practice, I hear the '90s hip hop song by Black Sheep that opens with the choice of one option … or another. The repetition of this phrase over and over, just like the song intro, is exactly what it feels like in the mind of a person who needs this flower essence. Scleranthus supports us when we are faced with an important decision but paralyzed with fear or anxiety. In this state, we go back and forth between our options, gather way too much information, and ask for advice from everyone who will listen. Yet, we still cannot make up our minds.

Scleranthus is indicated when we have trouble making minor decisions: "Should I wear the red shirt or the blue shirt? Should I take the train or the bus? Should I drive or should I carpool? Should I have chicken or fish for dinner?" We find ourselves going back and forth in our minds deciding between really mundane things. But often underlying seemingly insignificant choices is a big life decision on the horizon. "Which college should I go to?" "Should I leave my husband or stay in this marriage?" "Is now the right time to have a baby?" These are decisions for which there is no clear right or wrong, and the options are equally weighted. At these crossroads, we intuitively know that the choice we make will change our life.

We need Scleranthus flower essence when we are pretty freaked out, afraid that we are one decision away from total ruin. Scleranthus brings a sense of calm clarity, helping us to trust ourselves. We are able to listen to our intuition and make a decision to move forward. Scleranthus helps us trust that we are following the path that is right for us. It moves us out of paralysis and the fear of ruining our lives, cultivates a sense of calm knowing that we can change our minds if we need to. We feel supported in knowing that no matter what, we will be OK. We feel the support of the spiritual realm, that will benevolently guide us back to ourselves rather than punish us. There is no wrong answer. Once we make an executive decision, we move forward with clarity to receive the lessons and blessings that come from pursuing our purpose.

Blackberry: Take Action—Blackberry flower essence helps us get busy when we're stuck in procrastination and lethargy, and when we are talking the talk more than we're actually walking the walk. It is the quintessential essence to help us manifest our ideas through concrete actions to make it happen. I call Blackberry the "don't talk about it, BE about it!" flower essence.

The Wood element supports forward movement and personal evolution. When our Wood element is activated, we are flooded with creative ideas and vision. If we're not careful, we can mistake the ideas and vision for the action.

Our dreams stay in our imagination without becoming reality. Blackberry helps us take the first steps we need to bring our vision to life. Sometimes the sheer magnitude of our vision can overwhelm us. We have a detailed to-do list, and everything on that list is equally important and urgent. What ends up getting done is nothing because we're so busy thinking about all the things that we have to do that we don't do any of them. Blackberry helps us break through this paralysis and procrastination.

What I love about Blackberry flower essence is that it helps us take the steps instead of just thinking about them. One of my clients had a beautiful vision for a wellness practice. It completely aligned with her destiny, but she didn't know where to start. She had been dreaming about this practice for about two years before we began working together, and she was beginning to doubt if she had what it took to realize this dream. Within two weeks of working with Blackberry, she had a breakthrough. She called to let me know that she had registered her business, filed the LLC paperwork, opened a business bank account, and had commissioned a graphic designer to create her logo—all within the same week! Blackberry helped her realize that there was nothing to it but to do it. Rather than being overwhelmed by the greatness of her vision, she was able to see and take the small steps that would get her to her goal.

No matter the task in front of us, Blackberry helps to break it into smaller, actionable steps. Instead of thinking about our to-do list over and over, we make the call, press the button, take the step. Blackberry heightens our awareness that thinking about a task *and* doing it can actually happen at the same time. As we cross things off of our checklist, we feel the sense of agency and accomplishment that are signatures of a healthy Wood element.

Embodied Practice: Vrikshasana (Tree Pose)

Affirmation: I root, I rise.

From a standing position, shift your weight onto your left foot. Envision the roots growing out of the sole of your foot, anchoring you to the earth. When you have your balance, slowly bend your right knee and place the sole of your foot on your inner left ankle or shin, or above the left knee.

Clasp your hands together above your head, releasing the index fingers to point directly above you. Look up toward your fingertips. Feel a stretch in two directions: anchoring into the earth yet expanded toward the sky.

Close your eyes and imagine that you are a sprout, unapologetically reaching for the sun. Repeat the affirmation: *I root, I rise.*

Relax your arms and legs, and repeat on the opposite side.

Music Is Medicine: Playlist for the Wood Element

Use your Wood element playlist whenever you need confidence, motivation, or to get up and at 'em! The songs below express the archetypal signatures and sounds of the Wood element. Many in this list have explicit lyrics; by the time folks get to cussin', usually the Wood element is involved! Enjoy but... maybe not around the kiddos.

"Green Garden" by Laura Mvula
Album: Sing to the Moon, RCA Victor, 2013

The color of the Wood element is green, and its season is spring when the plant world emerges from the darkness of winter. So not only does "Green Garden" literally reference the Wood element, it also energetically conveys the freedom and ease the Wood element gifts us. This element brings us contentment and satisfaction, a smile on the inside that knows all is right in the world. This song puts me right in that space each and every time.

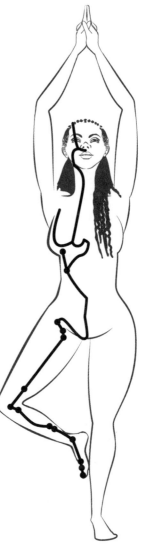

Pictured with
the Liver Meridian

"Scale" by Winter Flags
Album: Winter Flags, Dado Records, 2013

This song by Winter Flags needs no words to convey the hope and aspiration that a healthy Wood element offers. The rising, climbing melody is a signature for the Wood's constant striving for success, and the perseverance to reach our for the Wood's constant striving for success, and the perseverance to reach our goals. When are living on purpose and walking our destined path, we also feel a sense of ease and contentment that this song evokes. One of the most popular herbs in Chinese Medicine for treating the Wood element is translated as "free and easy wanderer." When our path and vision is clear, life feels effortless and free!

"Level Up" by Ciara
Album: Beauty Marks, *Beauty Marks Entertainment, 2019*

The energetic of the Wood element is up…all the way up! The metaphor for the Wood element is the sprout and the tremendous upward energy it takes to counter the force of gravity and burst through the soil. The Wood element inspires us to be at the top of our game, as we strive to self-actualize and bring the best of ourselves into the world. Entrepreneurship and artistic creativity also fall under the Wood element's domain. When the Wood element is healthy, we rise to the challenge of making sure our unique brilliance is respected. There's no limit to how high we can go!

"Blessed" by Shenseea featuring Tyga
Album: Blessed, *Rich Immigrants/Interscope Records, 2019*

Listen. If you ever need a confidence-boosting, Wood-element-inspired way to start your day, this song is it! Shenseea chants about her unapologetic greatness without forgetting to shout out her blessings. When we are bold enough to declare ourselves invincible and "unfuckwitable," we know that the Wood element is not far behind us.

"Middle Child" by J. Cole
Album: Revenge of the Dreamers III,
Dreamville/Roc Nation/Interscope, 2019

The Wood element evokes the archetype of the Champion, just like this anthem by J. Cole. When our Wood element is activated, we are determined to win and willing to put in the work to make it to the top. This song reflects the Wood element's tenacity, determination, and drive.

"Soldier" by Erykah Badu
Album: New Amerykah Part One (4th World War),
Universal Motown/Control Freaq, 2008

Erykah Badu is known for being eccentric and revolutionary, which are qualities of a healthy Wood element. The Gallbladder, the organ associated with the Wood element, is also called "the General", so the militaristic march of "Soldier" earns its spot on this playlist. The Wood element also governs social justice and equality—everyone should have the right to resources. In "Soldier," Erykah inspires us to stay woke to and take a stand for our rights.

"Dispear" by Nas and Damian Marley
Album: Distant Relatives, *Universal Republic/Def Jam Recordings, 2010*

Speaking of military vibe, next on the list we come to "Dispear." An archetype of the Wood element is the Warrior, especially the Spiritual Warrior. Between the evocation of ancestral warriors and the rhythmic war cry, this song transports me to past lives putting on war paint while preparing for battle. And in typical Wood element fashion, Nas's voice and lyrics cut unflinchingly straight to the point.

"Mad" by Solange featuring Lil Wayne
Album: A Seat at the Table, *Saint/Columbia Records, 2016*

What happens when the natural upward movement of the soul gets blocked? What happens when we are denied the right to express ourselves and stand in our power? Righteous indignation, a.k.a anger or even rage. Though the emotion has a bad reputation, it's really the appropriate response to the violations of the self. The trick is learning to respond with consequences and boundaries. When we learn to appropriately respond to our triggers, rather than merely exploding or imploding, anger can be a powerful catalyst for growth and change.

"Caught Out There" by Kelis
Album: Kaleidoscope, *Virgin Records, 1999*

OK, this is Wood gone really, really, really wrong. The emotion associated with the Wood element is anger and its many manifestations, from minor irritability to full-blown rage. It's especially loud when there's pent-up resentment and frustration that stem from the inability to make a change. Enter Kelis and all this madness. If ever you should find yourself trashing the house screaming "AAHHHGGG!" (and who hasn't been *there*?) then I suggest you flip back through these pages and get some soul medicine for the Wood element. I'm just sayin'.

"This Is America" by Childish Gambino
Single, McDJ/RCA Records, 2018

Speaking of war, Childish Gambino is stirred up controversy with his video for "This Is America," in which a gospel choir is ruthlessly gunned down. Whether we love or hate the video, I don't think we can deny Mr. Glover's unflinching gaze at American policy, channeling the Wood element's ability to question, confront, and transform. I'm particularly struck by the symbolism in the video representing the struggle to make #BlackLivesMatter in a country where, historically, they don't.

"Time 4 Sum Aksion" by Redman
Album: Whut? Thee Album, *Def Jam Recordings, 1993*

Let's get ready to ruuummmmble! The Wood element is about taking concrete action in the world—*now*. When the Wood element is blocked, we feel stuck in procrastination or an endless cycle of ideas that never manifest. But when the Wood element is thriving, we experience an eruption of clear intention along with the energy and motivation to make it happen.

Beychella

If you haven't had a chance to watch Beyoncé's killer performance at Coachella, please dedicate two hours of your life to this incredible homage to Black music. Beychella and the documentary *Homecoming* make the Wood element list not only because Bey is truly at the top of her game but because she uses her art to stand unapologetically in her self-definition. Her rendition of "Lift Every Voice" following "Formation" made me so proud, and I loved her cheeky side-eye at Coachella for being the first Black woman to headline. Looking at her catalog, we can truly get a sense of Bey's evolution over time, which is what the Wood element is all about.

"Tomorrow (A Better You, Better Me)" by Quincy Jones featuring Tevin Campbell
Album: Back on the Block, Qwest/Warner Bros, 1989

Sung by teen sensation Tevin Campbell, this song channels the youthful energy of the Wood element. The last acupuncture point on the Liver meridian is called the Gate of Hope. The Wood element brings us not only hope but also a vision for the future to strive toward. It helps us reconcile the tension between peace and passivity in the struggle against oppression. Just as the sun rises and shines anew, this song offers the gentle, inspired hope that tomorrow will be better.

Wood in Practice: Reaction versus Response

The Wood element teaches us that anger is healthy and appropriate in some situations, and we are responsible for how that anger is expressed. If we rage out of control or shrink from confrontation, our integrity is compromised. But more importantly, as far as the Wood element is concerned, nothing changes.

I coach my clients to think about anger in two phases: the reaction, and the response. The reaction is what moves qi and flows with an energy determined to rise. We might yell, curse, hit, or break things (not healthy), or journal, exercise, or throw eggs in the shower (much healthier). The point is that all responses move the qi but none of them tend to create any kind of change. Have you ever yelled like a maniac at someone who *still* did not listen to what you said? It's pretty maddening, but it happens all the time.

Your reaction (or lack thereof) is only half of the anger = change equation. The second half is your response. While the reaction is a powerful way to move your Wood element qi, it's the response that actually facilitates the change. The Wood element's lesson is that we need to both respond *and* react. The clearer we are on why our anger was triggered in the first place, the more capable we are of asserting change.

Use the following chart to process your anger cues:

Anger = Change

Scenario

When was the last time you felt anger or one of its forms—rage, irritation, or frustration?

React

How did you react? What did you do or say (with your words AND your body language?)

Signal

What was your anger a singal for?
+ Unaddressed issue
+ Self-compromise (ignoring your own needs)
+ Overextension of self (doing or giving more than you should)
+ Competence/growth restricted
+ Freedom obstructed
+ Boundaries violated

Respond

What can you put in place to address the real issue? Who can help?

Re-Reaction

If this situation happens again, what can you do differently?

Chapter 5
Dancing Fire

In our modern world, we no longer rely on fire for light or heat. More often than not, we use it to set a mood. We light candles on birthday cakes to celebrate life. We may plan a romantic candlelit dinner, or light candles in our bedrooms for sexy vibes. We light candles on our altars for prayer or meditation and during healing treatments to help us focus inward. All of these moments highlight the Fire element's role, which helps us celebrate life and experience sexual, emotional, and spiritual intimacy.

Fire Element Signatures

We can recognize the archetypal qualities of the Fire element through the following signatures:

- Season: Summer
- Phase: Flower
- Color: Red
- Energetic: Scatters and expands qi
- Core Emotions: Love, joy
- Sound: Laughing
- Meridians: Heart, Small Intestine, Triple Heater

Season: Summer
In the Wood element, you are striving for the sun; in the Fire element, you *are* the sun. Summer is the season of the Fire element. In the summer, flowers blossom into their unique beauty and glory, just as our Fire element governs our ability to shine our uniqueness into the world. Summer is alive and vibrant as we connect with our friends and head outdoors. Our joy is contagious.

Phase: Flower

Since we are halfway through the cycle of the elements, let's do a quick recap of each phase using the example of starting a business. Water, the incubation phase, is when you have your idea. The seed is planted. In Wood, the sprout, you clarify your vision and start actively taking steps to achieve you goal. When you get to Fire, you're like, "Here I am! Look what I'm up to!" You post on social media, create flyers and newsletters, network, and start attracting potential clients or collaborators.

The Fire element marks the phase when things start to blossom and take on a life of their own. The love within our hearts swells or our projects reach their zenith, and we become ready to share and celebrate with others. Just like a flower, things shine, radiate, and attract in the Fire element phase. Fire gifts us with the ability to magnetically draw things to us like a moth to a flame. In the Fire phase of any process, you show up to be revealed, witnessed, and celebrated.

Color: Red

In Classical Five Element acupuncture, the color of the Fire element is red. This is the bright red of vibrant flowers such as peonies and zinnias, or the spicy red of a ripe pepper or tomato. Fire is reflected in the deep red of our blood, and the striking red of a cardinal's wings. We also see Fire's red in the bright pink of a baby's tongue, the warm golden red of a sunset, and the archetypal red hearts associated with Valentine's Day.

Energetic: Scatters and Expands Qi

Just as the Water element brings us to our depths, the Fire element brings us to our heights. Fire is the most yang of all elements, bringing with it energy, spirit, and dynamic movement.

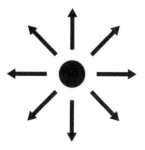

The energetic of the Fire element is outward expansion, just as fireworks explode and light up the night sky. Fireworks move from the center out to the periphery, just like love. Fire teaches us how to ignite the spark within ourselves, and then to shine that love out into the world. Fire is our energetic capacity to shine and expand.

Another thing about Fire—it knows how to turn up! When out of balance, the uber-excitement of Fire scatters our qi just like a firework. Here's an example: a few weeks ago, I visited my mom and met her new puppy, Cole. Let me tell you, Cole greeted every morning ready to press the Go! button. I would let him out of his doggy bed at 6:30 a.m., and he would run around the room at least four times in excitement. He was so unable to contain himself that he would sometimes run into things and nearly knock himself out. When we feel ungrounded and "all over the place," we can suspect that the Fire element is highly activated. I call this out of control feeling the Wild Fire. Wild Fire is the mania of a child without a nap who's had way too much sugar. Wild Fire is the packed schedule and fitting more into a day than even the longer hours of sunlight can accommodate. Wild Fire is the creative burst that makes us skip meals and stay up all night because we are flooded with inspiration. Wild Fire is the puppy love that makes us ignore the red flags in a budding relationship. Wild Fire can also make us addicted to substances, experiences, or people who bring us pleasure.

Core Emotions: Love, Joy

In its natural expression, the Fire element is warm and radiant. Take a moment to think about someone you love and care for. Where do you feel that love in your body? Perhaps you feel a gentle, radiating warmth in your heart center. Take a moment to sense how those loving feelings move your qi.

Now think of someone you are experiencing conflict with. How does that heart-centered feeling shift? Rather than "up and out," perhaps you noticed that the warm fuzzies you felt a moment ago now feel tense, locked, or closed off. Working with the Fire element can help us restore the organic flow of our heart center.

To understand the Fire element, take two candles and hold them close to one another. The flames each flicker in their own independent dance. As you draw the two flames closer together, they seem to reach for one another, yearning to merge. When they finally touch, there is an orgasmic spark as they become one flame, shining even brighter as their lights become inseparable. When you pull the candles apart, they become individual flames again, content in their private dances.

Just like these candles, the Fire element teaches about the ecstatic and orgasmic joy of union. Fire is present in any moment where sparks fly! We can experience that spark in many ways: sexual orgasm, a spiritual a-ha moment or epiphany, engaging in something we feel passionate about, or that moment when you feel completely seen and understood by someone you love. When Fire is in the room, we feel elevated with the joy and excitement of connection.

The Fire element is also there to support us when those metaphorical candles pull apart. What happens when I can't do what I love doing? What happens when I can't be with a person that I love? What happens when my relationships end? The Fire element not only guides us as our hearts experience our fullest capacity for connection and joy, it is also there to teach us how to fuel our own inner flame in the face of heartache.

The Fire element is present in all relationships—romantic, sexual, familial, social, professional, and spiritual. Fire supports varying degrees of intimate connection as well as the boundaries we put into place to protect this most vulnerable aspect of ourselves. We can call on Fire to help us heal any of the blocks that keep us from experiencing our natural ability to form healthy connections. These blocks may be the leftovers from a painful breakup, sexual trauma, or any kind of physical or emotional abuse.

Listed here are several emotions that are moved by the Fire element:

Joy	Ecstasy	Pleasure
Love	Compassion	Adoration
Self-Doubt	Insecurity	Mania
Anxiety	Dissociation	Depression
Discouragement	Betrayal	Shame
Heartache	Loneliness	Rejection

Sound: Laughing

The sound of the Fire element in a person's voice is "laughing," with highs and lows that are spontaneous, animated, or excited. You can hear a laughing voice by giggling to yourself as you exclaim, "This is the best day of my life!" You can tell when Fire is in the room when a person sounds like there is a smile in their voice, even and especially when they share something they are not happy about. In fact, a strong Fire element might make a person smile or laugh to mask deeper, more uncomfortable feelings.

In music, the Fire element shows up in any song that conveys the deeply felt emotions of the heart. Music with sensual rhythms that inspire sexual intimacy and expression are also Fire in nature, including SOCA and dancehall. You can look at the Billboard top hits for any genre in any year and you will likely find some poignant love songs at the top of the list to stoke your Fire. Ecstatic trance music such as house, techno, drum & bass, and African drums resonate with the heartbeat and with the Fire element. (I've watched house dancers at the Soul Summit in Brooklyn, convinced that they might leave their body at any minute and levitate toward the sun.) Your Fire element playlist will include music that helps you feel joyful, energized, sexy, or loving.

Meridians: Heart, Small Intestine, Pericardium, Triple Heater

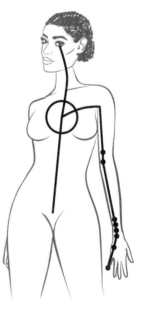

The Fire element is the only element that has two pairs of yin and yang meridians. The first set, the Heart and Small Intestine meridians, are related to the joy that comes from the union within oneself. This aspect of Fire supports our connection to our divinity and to our spiritual source.

The Heart Meridian [**Figure 5.1**] runs along the inner arm, with an internal branch that encircles the heart, dances across the chest, and connects to the eyes. The Small Intestine [**Figure 5.2**] travels along the outer arm, shoulders, upper back, and neck before ending in the inner ear. These two paired meridians are responsible for the complementary muscle systems required for healthy posture. When

5.1 Heart Meridian

someone is feeling sad, lacking confidence, or going through a hard time in a relationship, posture slumps. They may cave the back inward and slouch, as if protecting their heart. As a person moves through their healing with the Fire element, their posture will shift to reflect a vertical pole from Heaven to Earth.

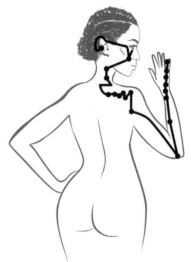

One of my favorite books to inspire my Fire element is hilarious self-help memoire *Year of Yes: How to Dance It Out, Stand in the Sun, and Be Your Own Person* (five points if you can list all the Fire element signatures in that book title!). Let me tell you, I laughed so hard reading this book on the train that people got up and moved two seats away from me! In one of the chapters, Shonda talks about her personal discovery of the relationship between her posture and her confidence. She writes:

5.2 Small Intestine Meridian

> Power posing like Wonder Woman is when you stand up like a bad-ass—legs in a wide stance, chin up, hands on your hips. Like you own the place. Like you have on magical silver bracelets and know how to use them. Like your superhero cape is flapping in the wind behind you…
>
> [A]ctual studies say that power posing like Wonder Woman for five minutes not only improves self-esteem but even hours later improves how other perceive you.

Let me say that again.

> *Standing around like Wonder Woman in the morning can make people think you are more amazing at lunchtime.*"[50]

Shonda ain't lying. Several studies in the field of psychophysiology explore the interconnection between posture, mood and cognition. One study demon-

---

50. Shonda Rhimes, *Year of Yes: How to Dance It Out, Stand in the Sun and Be Your Own Person* (Waterville, ME: Thorndike Press, 2016).

strated that hopeless, helpless, and powerless memories surface more readily in a slouched position and are accompanied by hormonal changes that contribute to increased stress, anxiety, and depression.[51] Another clinical study found that the surface electromyography of the upper trapezius, medial, and anterior deltoid muscles were significantly higher when in an erect posture as compared to in a slouched position.[52] Students in San Francisco State University conducted research to prove that straightening a collapsed posture into an assertive power posture leads to calmer and clearer thinking.[53] If you ever needed validation of taking your Wonder Woman stance in their world, science has your back.

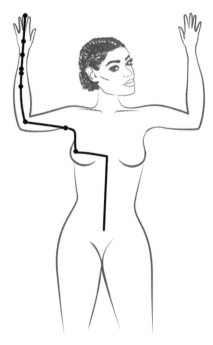

5.3 Pericardium Meridian

The second set of meridians for the Fire element include the Pericardium and the Triple Heater. The Heart and Small Intestine meridians carry the consciousness to help us connect to our authentic Self and the divine. Clinically, I turn to the Pericardium and Triple Heater meridians to support our ability to form healthy connections with one another.

In the human body, the pericardium looks like a sac that envelops the heart. It is a semi-permeable membrane, which means it lets some things in and keeps other things out. I imagine it like a window screen—fresh breeze in, mosquitoes out. In the same way, it helps us navigate heart-centered boundaries in

51. Vietta E. Wilson and Erik Peper, "The Effects of Upright and Slumped Postures on the Recall of Positive and Negative Thoughts," *Applied Psychophysiology and Biofeedback* 29, no. 3 (2004): 189–195.

52. Erik Peper et al., "Increase Strength and Mood with Posture," *Biofeedback* 44, no. 2 (January 2016): 66–72.

53. Ibid.

our relationships. When I feel a fluttering on the Pericardium pulse, I suspect that a person is navigating feelings of vulnerability. This aspect of the Fire element is also useful for treating feelings of betrayal, heartache, and distrust.

When we hold our arms so that the Pericardium meridian is facing the world, we hold a position of extraordinary vulnerability. [**Figure 5.3**] In the wake of increased police brutality, I felt triggered on my morning neighborhood runs. Dressed in my hoodies and athletic gear, I would raise my hands into plain sight when I passed police officers to not be mistaken for a Black man running in the streets, which might have had deadly consequences. This "Hands Up, Don't Shoot" posture conveys that we have no armor or weapon, and pleads that our essential humanity be seen, witnessed, and respected.

Our modern, technological society invites us out of the natural environment and into a world that involves countless hours on a computer. Many of us develop unhealthy postural habits, from extensive computer use, cell phone texting, and interacting through devices that make our posture slump into a permanent C curve. In a collapsed posture, the Heart meridian in the front of the body is compressed while the Small Intestine meridian is stretched out of proper proportion. The COVID-19 pandemic, which required many to work and attend school from home, has had an extraordinary impact on physical and emotional well-being, including increased feelings of helplessness, anxiety, isolation, and sadness. Sitting in a slouched position can create—or reflect—a blockage in the Fire element meridians.

Symptoms of Fire element disharmony include:

+ Insomnia
+ Anxiety
+ Heart Palpitations
+ Chest Pain
+ Vivid Dreams
+ Emotional Instability
+ Unexplained Sadness
+ Poor/Collapsed posture

There's an old wellness adage that says, "Dieting is for the body, exercise is for the mind." The Fire element governs the heart, which perceives and processes all emotions. Any cardiovascular exercise that gets the heart pumping—dance, running, swimming, cycling, and even sex—will nourish the Fire element and allow the heart to access emotional clarity. Bringing awareness of expansion and movement from the heart center will enliven any yoga pose with Fire's signature. As the meridians of the Fire element also traverse the upper back and shoulder blades, postures that stretch and benefit the shoulders also benefit Fire. Backbends that allow the heart to lift and expand are beneficial to Fire. In many cases, these postures can spark the awareness or release of the many emotions that the heart is holding.

The series of yoga postures in this chapter stretch and energize the Fire element meridians, and counteract the negative impact of sitting at a desk as well as the emotional impact of isolation. The exercises lengthen and relax the muscles of the shoulders, chest, and back to align our posture. However, the true magic of these poses is that they activate the Fire element so that we can feel reconnected, energized, calm, and clear.

Soul Lesson 1: You Are Whole

You don't need another person, place or thing to make you whole.
God already did that. Your job is to know it.
—*Maya Angelou*

Fire governs the spirit, and the light of divinity within us. It brings us the spark of insight and awareness that keeps us connected to our spiritual source. Fire gifts us with self-awareness and integrity, giving us the ability to act in alignment with our truest selves. In the face of external physical, emotional, psychic, or spiritual stress, Fire represents the light of the true self shining through.

Chinese Medicine offers a beautiful cosmic creation story that helps us to understand this aspect of the Fire element. In the beginning, there was nothing. Or rather, there was everything. The entire cosmos was interconnected as a single entity, representing complete oneness and unity. Then there was a grand explosion, a huge firework of the entire universe. Each spark of that explosion became a new soul. This spark is the *shen*, and we each carry this divine spark of the entire universe in our hearts.

The Chinese character for the word "heart," expressed as *xīn* in pinyin, is depicted as a bowl with a little spark in it. This spark may have been one of most ancient representations of shen. Though the word *shen* is specific to Chinese Medicine and philosophy, the concept of our essential divinity exists in many religious teachings. Some of us refer to this spark as our higher self; others call it our Christ Consciousness. In African spirituality, the concept closely resembles the Ori, or the spiritual guide the aligns each person with their unique purpose. No matter what we name this in our religious or spiritual practices, our connection to this spark allows us to navigate our lives successfully. When we are in touch with this spark, we love freely and fully. We're able to live in our purpose. We're able to follow our destiny. We're able to know what's right for us. We're able to know what we need. The Fire element teaches us how to remain connected to this spark in our hearts.

Classical Chinese Medicine texts tell us that that the primary responsibility of the Fire element is "housing the spirit," or the shen: "The Shen enables people to radiate outwards. Shen gives a person a sparkle in the eyes, inner vitality, joie de vivre, and an alertness of the mind."[54] When the Fire element is imbalanced, we experience feelings of disconnection, anxiety, sadness, and confusion. When healthy, we can problem solve, think creatively, and have a sense of purpose and assuredness. When we are connected to our shen, we are guided by an inner compass.

When someone is excited and their eyes sparkle, that's their shen. When we stare deeply and romantically into a lover's eyes, we are connecting with their shen. Shen is like the pilot light for our being. Its warm, steady presence helps us to light up every other aspect of our life.

In the mythology of Chinese Medicine, it is said that little red birds act as custodians of the divine spark. These shen birds fly up to the sun to receive the messages from the Divine during the day. At night, the birds return and rest in our hearts, where they share those messages from Heaven through our dreams and intuition. But when life gets too messy here on Earth, the shen birds fly the coop, taking our divine spark and hanging out in the heavens until it is safe to come back and settle in our hearts. Thousands of years ago, this metaphor was used to describe the symptoms that we now attribute to trauma and Post-Traumatic Stress Disorder (PTSD). The symbolic meta-

---

54. Angela Hicks, John Hicks, and Peter Mole, *Five Element Constitutional Acupuncture* (Edinburgh, UK: Churchill Livingstone, 2011), 89.

phor of the shen birds is clinically relevant: Heart palpitations often feel like a wild bird fluttering in the chest. When someone feels disassociated, they often describe their experiences as if watching their life from a bird's-eye view. Other symptoms of shen disturbance include anxiety, insomnia, wild dreams, difficulty with making decisions, feeling disconnected, and excessive daydreaming.

Our hearts take the hits from the curveballs life throws at us. An unexpected conflict, emotional or physical assault, the end of a relationship, a job loss, death of a loved one, and even prolonged periods of unrelenting stress—any situation that makes us gasp—all have the potential to scatter the Heart's qi, sending those shen birds flying, and thus extinguishing our pilot lights. If you've ever worked with a gas stove, you know what happen when the pilot light is out. You can turn up the gas all the way, but nothing happens. The same is true of the divine spark, or shen, as the pilot light of our souls. It doesn't matter what we experience—the most loving person, the most joyous trip, the biggest adventure—if that pilot light is out, there's nothing to catch fire. There is no spark to ignite our passion and joy.

The beauty of this philosophy is that no matter what we experience, nothing can damage or destroy shen, the aspect of our being that connects us to the Divine. Worst-case scenario, those shen birds hit us with a peace sign and roll out with our divine spark to keep it safe, or the pilot light needs a boost to reignite. But even in the face of the worst traumas and heartaches, our spirit remains perfect. Healing with the Fire element is not about fixing something broken. Rather, Fire teaches us how to reconnect to that part of ourselves that is connected to the entire universe. Fire reminds us that even when we feel broken, we are whole.

Reflection Questions

Are you connected to your inherent wholeness? Take a moment to reflect on the following questions in your journal:

+ When do you most feel like yourself?
+ Can you think of a time you felt like you were living someone else's life?
+ Who or what do you turn to when you need encouragement?
+ What heals your heart when it feels broken?

- Have you ever hit "rock bottom"? If so, what did it feel like?
- What healing resources are around you to address any unresolved wounds or traumas?

Flower Essence for Wholeness

The following flower essences help us reestablish a sense of wholeness and well-being:

- Star of Bethlehem for realignment with our self
- Echinacea for restoration of the self
- Deerbrush for heart and mind integrity

Star of Bethlehem: Realignment with Our Self—When you make eye contact with even a stranger, there is a subtle spark of recognition, acknowledgment, or warmth. But when someone we love has lost connection to their shen, it's as if there's no spark. That person may have a hard time making eye contact with you or holding your gaze. Or when you do look in their eyes, there's no life that comes back to you. You can't connect with them and get the sense that even though their body is right in front of you, the light of their soul is entirely somewhere else.

I saw a lot of patients and high school students with disturbed shen at the beginning of COVID. I could feel the vacancy and despair even through the screens of our virtual classes. Adults and teens alike were expressing the same sentiments: "I don't know what to do with my life, I don't feel passionate about anything." "Everything just kind of feels blocked." When we are disconnected from our shen, we may go through the motions, doing the things we always do but without finding any joy or pleasure in them. The spark is gone.

Star of Bethlehem is the flower essence we call on for any type of shock—the unexpected death of a loved one, a divorce or breakup, any kind of betrayal, or a physical accident. Anything in our lives that makes us do a double-take and ask ourselves, "What just happened?!" can disrupt our connection with our shen. Star of Bethlehem is the first flower I turn to for acute trauma, heartache, or even prolonged emotional stress. It is useful for the symptoms associated with a rattled shen: overwhelm, anxiety, disassociation, a feeling being off-centered and unable to recalibrate. It settles the shen back into the heart.

I also use it to "reignite the pilot light" that can be blown out by overwhelming experiences.

I once had a client who was doing a lot of intense spiritual work. He shared that he could not relate or connect to the many blessings and opportunities surrounding him. He felt like an observer, standing outside of himself as he witnessed his life happening to someone else. He also suffered from terrible nightmares, which made him feel even less grounded. During the consultation, he had a difficult time sustaining eye contact with me. These were all signs that the shen birds had taken flight. With Star of Bethlehem flower essence, he was able to gradually come back into alignment and to experience himself as an actual participant in his life.

It was the Star of Bethlehem shining brightly in the night sky that led the three Wise Men to the Christ child. The legend tells us that once the magi arrived, the star completed its purpose. It then burst into thousands of pieces, and each piece that fell to Earth became one of the beautiful, white star-shaped flowers known as Star of Bethlehem.

Just as the luminous star guided the wise men, the Star of Bethlehem flower essence guides us back to ourselves. It realigns us with our true north. And just as the fragments of the star's explosion became a beautiful flower, our individual shen is a spark of the explosion of the divine cosmos. The similarities between these two stories, although from different spiritual traditions, give us insight into the role that Star of Bethlehem plays in reconnecting us to our divine spark that lives in our hearts. It is the flower essence to call on whenever we need to be reminded of the divine nature, purpose, and unfolding of our lives.

Echinacea: Restoration of the Self—Also called purple coneflower, echinacea is one of the most widely used herbal remedies. Though it has many uses, it is most commonly used during cold and flu season as an immunity booster, and studies have shown that it increases our white blood cell count to fight off disease. To understand how Echinacea works as a flower essence, we have to know a little bit about our miraculous immune system.

Our immune system works something like this: We have a community of cells working in beautiful harmony to carry out the functions of our bodies—breathing, sleeping, eating, dreaming, dancing, to name a few. Imagine that our body is like having the best party in the universe. Every now and then, someone uninvited wants in on the action and tries to crash the party. In Western medicine, we call this party crasher a virus, bacteria, or germ.

Our immune system is the bouncer standing at the door of the party. They check IDs, tell the virus, "sorry bub, you're not invited" and send them on their way. But sometimes the virus manages to get past the bouncer and then lets all their friends in the back door. So now, the viruses are in the party (our body) having a good ol time. But because they are haters and don't really belong, they start messing up things. They knock over the DJ, insult the guests, and before you know it, the party isn't so great. We call this getting sick. Now, it takes some time for the bouncers to find all of these party crashers and get them out. And the longer they were in there running amok, the more repair we'll need before the party can start feeling like a party again.

As an herbal medicine, Echinacea is the look-out that calls more bouncers so that a) fewer crashers get in and b) they don't hang out as long if they do get in. Echinacea flower essence does the same thing on a psychic and emotional level. Echinacea is indicated when the person's sense of self and integrity are disrupted. Physical and emotional stress and trauma and stress weaken our psychic and emotional defenses. As a result, negative thoughts and ideas sneak in as viruses and take over the party. Sometimes these gangsters hang out for so long, we don't even realize they weren't invited. We accept negative beliefs about ourselves and our self-worth without questioning them, and the party isn't what it should be. Echinacea flower essence calls in a backup security team to help restore the party to its original greatness. As a result, we feel in alignment with ourselves again and in touch with our essential dignity.

I use Echinacea flower essence whenever a client has suffered from prolonged emotional distress or a physical trauma such as a car accident or surgery. I also use Echinacea when deep shame prevents a person from seeing their own greatness, advocating for themselves, or connecting to their divine spark. Often (but not always), this is a result of abuse, neglect, or a devastating circumstance. Echinacea is useful for my clients who work in oppressive environments where constant microaggressions over time wear down even the strongest sense of dignity and esteem. Echinacea is also helpful for someone actively recovering from an abusive situation or addiction (with the help of a licensed professional), as it helps to us to re-constellate when our sense of our core identity that has been shattered.

Deerbrush: Heart and Mind Integrity—Deerbrush is a cluster flower that looks like little white soap suds that cleanse and reveal desires of the heart. There are many times when our hearts and our minds have two different ideas about what should go down. We feel confusion, anxiety, depression, and the many feelings that keep us from moving forward with clarity and conviction. Other times, we find ourselves saying or doing things that we can't explain. "Why did I just bug out? Why am I so mad?" "Why did I just sleep with this man I am clearly not interested in?" "Why did I just throw her shade?" When these questions are met with a dumbfounded shoulder shrug, it's time to call in Deerbrush flower essence.

Deerbrush is also helpful when the stress is so overwhelming that we can't make simple decisions or be responsive to our own needs. When my uncle passed away last year, everyone swarmed around my cousin asking what she needed and what they could do to help. But she couldn't wrap her head around a coherent response because her mind was so consumed with caring for her grieving mother, funeral arrangements, and her upcoming licensing exams. Asking her to make one more decision seemed out of the question. I remember myself in similar states of overwhelm so bad that, ironically, even the adult coloring books I bought that were designed for relaxation created more anxiety! The stress of deciding about what color marker to use was more than I could handle. Working with Deerbrush helped me settle back into myself. It even led me and to discover the color-by-number books that I now swear by.

Integrity is at the core of Deerbrush, but what is integrity? Integrity comes when our feelings, actions, and words are in alignment. We mean what we say, and we say what we mean. There's no hidden agenda or passive aggressive shenanigans. Things are clear. But if we don't know, ignore, or numb how we feel, how can we find that alignment?

Traditional African and East Asian cultures speak of the intelligence of the heart. In Classical Chinese Medicine, the heart is considered the house of all of our emotions, our awareness, and intelligence. There are incredible similarities between the Chinese character and ancient Egyptian hieroglyphs for the heart, both which are depicted as a bowl or vessel. A better translation of the characters is heart-mind, because it is the heart that translates our feelings, experiences and information into meaning. Rather than considering the brain as the CEO, it is the heart charged with setting the agenda for our life. The heart has its own knowing. Deerbrush gives the heart-CEO's voice a seat at the table, and a position of authority.

The heart is a container for all emotions. In fact, as a symbolic language, the characters of all the emotions in Chinese writing contain the symbol for "heart," and when the heart is disturbed with tumultuous emotions, the spirit cannot rest. It's no coincidence that in ancient Kemetic philosophy, keeping one's heart as "light as a feather" is a central spiritual truth. Deerbrush helps clarify what our heart is holding, even emotions we are not consciously aware of. Is there hidden fear? Anger? Jealousy? Love? Deerbrush flower essence helps us to cultivate clarity and authenticity in our words, feelings, and actions.

Embodied Practice: Self-Hug

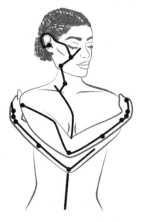

Affirmation: I am whole.

This pose can be done almost anywhere: sitting, standing, or lying in bed! Simply rest your hands on opposite shoulders and offer yourself a huge, warm hug. Close your eyes and gaze inward, or gaze into your eyes in a mirror. Imagine that you can see the original spark of the cosmos in your eyes, and radiating in your heart.

Repeat the affirmation:

In this moment, I am safe.

In this moment, I am whole.

In this moment, I am love.

**Pictured with the Small
Intestine Meridian**

Notice any internal dialogue that resists this moment of self-love and tenderness.

Soul Lesson 2: Open Your Heart

"Your task is not to seek for love, but merely to seek and find all
the barriers within yourself that you have built against it."
—Rumi

We use the language of Fire to describe the qualities of our relationships: When something warms our heart, we lean into emotional connection. Feeling "hot and bothered" means experiencing strong physical or sexual attraction. The people in our life who lack warmth and empathy are called cold-hearted. Without Fire's warmth, we have a hard time relating, socializing, and sustaining emotional or sexual connection.

Relationships light up something in our hearts and in our souls that allow us to feel more alive. Recent studies have shown that healthy relationships also significantly contribute to our physical and psychological well-being. Healthy relationships have been linked to increased immunity, cardiovascular health, and maintaining healthy weight. In addition to the physical benefits, relationships also help alleviate both short- and long-term stress. Researchers have found that a sense of social connection is linked to reduced anxiety and depression. In fact, one fascinating study by a psychologist at the University of Texas revealed that confiding in a trusted friend about a stressful event can improve immune function for as long as six months afterward.[55] I think about this study whenever I'm stressed, call a girlfriend, and immediately start feeling better after talking it out. Because we humans are social beings, relationships are a fundamental need, just as important as food, clothing, water, and shelter.

Perhaps we have all had the experience of being in a crowded room yet somehow still feeling alone. Our sense of loneliness does not stem from the number of people surrounding us but rather the sense of fulfillment we gain from our connections. In our increasingly social-media-heavy world, we could have ten thousand followers who like our posts but still don't cure our loneliness. The Fire element supports our capacity to form new healthy relationships and to experience a sense of fulfillment and connection within existing relationships.

---

55. James W. Pennebaker, *Opening Up: The Healing Power of Confiding in Others* (New York: William Morrow & Co., 1990).

We are so wired for connection that loneliness and isolation trigger the fight-or-flight stress response. Feelings of loneliness have been linked with neurological and hormone changes such as increased cortisol and inflammation. Loneliness also increases the risk for depression and suicide, antisocial behavior, decreased memory and learning, poor decision-making, and substance abuse.[56]

You would think that since relationships are so important to our health and well-being, they'd be easy, right? Nope! Relationship traumas and dramas are at the top of social media feeds, news stories, and reality TV. I can count on one hand the number of couples I know who are happily married, and even those couples unanimously agree that successful relationships are a lot of *work*, not to mention the stress and strain of family, friendships, and professional relationships. The Fire element teaches us not only how to have healthy relationships, but how to heal the wounds of love gone wrong.

When we hear the word "relationship," we often first think of intimate, romantic partners (which hints at the responsibility and expectation we often place on significant others). Our relationship needs can be met by romantic partnerships, as well as professional, family, spiritual, and social connections. What truly matters is our ability to have social ties that meet a variety of needs for belonging, support, and even physical touch. Fire teaches us how to find the balance between merging and separating without losing ourselves in any of those stages. Fire also teaches us how to be vulnerable enough to show up as our complete, whole selves.

In alchemy is the concept of something called a tempered fire, which is the exact temperature at which magic can happen. Take the alchemical art of cooking, for instance. Every chef knows that if the fire is too hot or too weak, things don't come out right. If I turn the flame too high, I'm going to burn the soup. It's going to stick to the bottom of the pan or evaporate too quickly. If there's not enough heat, all the ingredients are just going to sit in the pot without actually cooking—it'll basically be water with stuff floating in it. No thanks!

---

56. Keith J. Karren, N. Lee Smith, and Kathryn J Gordon, *Mind/Body Health: The Effects of Attitudes, Emotions, and Relationships* (Boston: Pearson, 2014), 263.

Building a relationship is like cooking a great soup. The Fire element teaches us how to keep the temperature just right so we can come together in the most beautiful way. The trick is monitoring that flame and turning things up or down as needed to make the magic happen. Maybe our relationship feels a little cold, distant, or stagnant. Time to turn up the heat! Send a spicy text or pic if it's a romantic relationship. Send a warm email to check in on a business partner if they seem to be dragging their feet on closing the deal. Offer a hug or compliment to the kid who seems a little distant. If things are moving too fast or with too much intensity, we want to cool those fires. This might mean taking a walk or getting some space to break up a heated argument. Or it might mean asking for additional time to feel into a decision that feels stressful and urgent. A "hakuna matata" style vacation—even if you don't leave your home—may be just what you need to cool down from an intense schedule.

Tempered fire is especially important when building new relationships. Having sex "too soon" or telling your deepest, darkest secrets on the first date might cause one or both partners to pull back (to balance out that intensity). The opposite can happen, too—after a week of date app texting with long gaps in between, there's just not enough heat to spark interest. The Fire element helps moderate the pace of what to conceal and reveal to create healthy emotional or physical intimacy.

Reflection Questions

What is the quality of your relationships? Take a moment to reflect on the following questions in your journal:

+ Which of your relationships are most valuable and meaningful?
+ Which of your relationships are a source of tension and conflict?
+ What are you learning about yourself through the significant relationships in your life?
+ What aspects of a relationship make it easy for you to trust or love open-heartedly?
+ Make a timeline of key relationships that stand out to you. What did you learn about love from these relationships?
+ Are there any of these lessons you need to unlearn to have more successful relationships?

Flower Essences to Open Your Heart

Use the flower essences below to expand your heart and support your relationships:

+ Holly to tear down walls around the heart
+ Chicory to fill with love from within
+ Spreading Phlox for soul-to-soul connection
+ Baby (Blue) Eyes to trust the world

Holly: Tear Down Walls—Holly is the first flower essence I turn to whenever there is any emotion that blocks the heart from connecting with others—especially fear, anger, or distrust. If we look at a holly flower, we see thick, waxy, thorny leaves protecting a delicate flower. The Fire element teaches us how to open our hearts to love, but that does not mean that our open hearts are a free-for-all. Instead, the Fire element teaches us the healthy discernment that we need to have appropriate boundaries in our relationships. We take responsibility for *who* and *how* we love.

From this perspective, Holly is the flower essence we call on when the Pericardium, or Heart Protector, is too rigid because of past hurts. The walls around the heart thicken with anger, jealously, or fear, making it impossible for true acceptance, love, and compassion to get in. Betrayal, suspicion and shame are also emotions that show up when the natural radiance of Fire element qi has been compromised. Holly offers first aid for the Fire element when we find ourselves looking through our lover's phone (I see you), armoring ourselves from emotional intimacy, and any of the ways we question our ability to love or be loved. These hardened emotions want to be a protective barrier, but in doing so, stifle the natural expression of the heart's joy from radiating outward.

Holly helps to nourish the heart's capacity for compassion and inner radiance, and supports us when we experience insecurity in both personal and professional relationships. Holly helps us radiate warmth and connection, helping the heart to open and trust that others are not going to cause harm. In professional relationships, it protects the heart when we are over-afraid that others will steal our ideas or sabotage our success.

Holly is an ally when we find ourselves holding on to past hurts, as well as when we withhold love, attention, and affection as subtle forms of punishment.

Holly is also indicated when we feel resentful or jealous due to not receiving enough love. It is equally useful for children experiencing sibling rivalry, puppies who must share their owners, and lovers who want more attention and affection from their partners. Holly warms the heart with loving magic and dissolves the walls of our heart so that the natural radiance of the Fire element can shine.

Chicory: Fill from Within—Chicory is classically prescribed for children who cry for attention through temper tantrums, showing off, displaying mean behavior, or whining and clinginess. If you've been around a child acting out to get your attention, you know what I'm talking about. But adults can act in the same way, being needy or clinging, acting mean and sulking, being loud and obnoxious, or having a full-on temper tantrum. The only real difference is that adults have more sophisticated language to justify their actions. But, the need for love, energy and attention is universal. When we really think about it, we all have our ways of "acting out" to get the love we crave.

For both children and adults, Chicory flower essence brings awareness to our patterns of manipulation. Perhaps we developed these patterns in childhood and carried them on into our adult lives. We might give someone the silent treatment or become passive aggressive when we don't feel like we can directly assert ourselves. We might feel needy and clingy in a way that is destructive to a relationship. We might become controlling or demanding for time, attention, and love. Chicory gently reminds us to ask ourselves, "What expectations do I have for others to fill a void within myself?" Chicory helps us to look inwardly at those patterns and helps us see what needs to be tweaked. This self-awareness allows us to bring more objectivity and integrity to our relationships.

The Celestine Prophecy by James Redfield offers a beautiful example of how Chicory can support the integrity of our relationships. In the story, a science teacher goes on a journey that teaches him about the energetic and metaphysical nature of the universe. Synchronicity helps him to be in the right place at the right time to uncover the nine insights of an ancient manuscript. In the fourth insight, he learns about "control dramas," which are the four key ways that people manipulate for energy in relationships. The four patterns are: the Intimidator, who bullies and demands attention by force; the Interrogator, who asks questions to draw a person out of themselves; the Aloof, who goes silent and cold, gaining attention by being mysterious; and the Poor Me, who plays the victim role to elicit attention in the form of sympathy. The Intimidator and Interrogator patterns both demand energy, while the Aloof and the Poor Me patterns assert that there is no energy to give. However, at the heart of it, all four patterns experience their own version of an energy deficit.[57]

These are just a few of the many maladaptive ways we try to relate to others. Perhaps you recognize some of these patterns in yourself, or in those you love? I certainly can. I tend to be an Interrogator. I don't even catch myself until I'm about five to ten questions in. Sometimes I'll realize that the person may be answering my questions, but we're not necessarily having a conversation. One night my daughter was being silent and withdrawn at dinner. I asked her questions about her school work, her teachers, her dance classes—anything and everything I thought might get her talking. Finally, she blew up and yelled, "I don't feel like being interviewed every night!" Let's just say dinner did not end well. In retrospect, I can see how our Chicory-needing behaviors were preventing authentic and meaningful connection. She was being Aloof, and I was being an Interrogator. Our patterns fed each other, and like the proverbial chicken and the egg, it's impossible to determine which came first.

In *The Celestine Prophecy*, the protagonist learns a Fire element lesson—how to reconnect to the spark of divinity as an ever-present source of love. He learns to go into nature, return to his breath, and feel complete within himself before trying to relate to others. Chicory helps us to cultivate what researchers call "creative solitude." Creative solitude helps us to cultivate an intimate relationship with our inner emotional landscape, instead of solely of seeking fulfillment from others. Hobbies such as journaling, gardening, creating art, learning a new language, writing, and playing a musical instrument all nurture the Fire element so that we can engage in relationships with our wholeness intact.

Chicory flower essence supports us feeling loved, complete, and supported from within. Once we are secure with the love within our own hearts, we approach our relationships with clarity and equanimity. Rather than compet-

---

57. James Redfield, *The Celestine Prophecy* (Hoover, AL: Satori Publishing, 1993), 235.

ing and manipulating for love, we learn to share love that overflows from the source and through our hearts.

Spreading Phlox: Soul-to-Soul Connection—Have you ever met someone and felt an instant and inexplicable connection to them? No doubt this person is part of your soul squad, a special tribe of folks who came down from the spirit world with you to help you fulfill your mission. When you find members of your soul squad, it can be very energizing! These folks might feel familiar, as if you've known them for lifetimes (you probably have).

I call Spreading Phlox the soul family flower, as it can be a catalyst for attracting the friends, intimate partners, and professional connections that we need to manifest our intentions for love and success. Spreading Phlox extends the forces of the heart center outward, so that we can call in or attract those with whom we have a karmic connection.

For example, Spreading Phlox opens us to the synchronicity thinking of a person whom you then just happen to run into. Or you tell the universe that you want to start painting, and the next thing you know, a casual conversation at the grocery store leads to you joining an art class that night. I offer Spreading Phlox to my clients who are beginning to date to help them call in their soul mates. Even the relationships that don't work out in the long run end up offering valuable lessons. Part of the subtle magic of how Spreading Phlox works is reconnecting us to those who are part of our journey and path. Spreading Phlox flower essence helps us to attract, meet, and form relationships with those who are meant to be part of our destiny, one way or another.

Sometimes the affection, ease, or intimacy in a relationship can be mistaken as a romantic attraction. Other times, we will feel put off by our tribe members as they trigger reminders of past wounds we need to heal. Our soul squad members teach us important life lessons, or reveal deeper truths that further us on our destined path. Whether they are meant to be in our lives for a reason, season, or a lifetime, Spreading Phlox helps us to connect us to our soul squad.

Baby (Blue) Eyes: Restore Trust—Imagine the most precious baby staring up you with innocence and wonder. They are close to the world of pure spirit and have not yet experienced the thorns of being human. They have not yet experienced disappointment or heartache, and have the full expectation that all of their needs will be met. Also called Baby Blue Eyes or Baby's-blue-eyes, *Nemophila menziesii* restores our trust in love and helps to dissolve the cynicism and armoring that form like scar tissue around a broken heart.

The flower does resemble a cluster of bright blue eyes staring upward to heaven. But before discussing its gifts, it's important to acknowledge that the name "Baby Blue Eyes" is steeped in Western Eurocentrism. The name is triggering for many people of color, including myself, because it suggests the perfect innocence of babies with blue eyes. I can remember clear as day when my second grade teacher announced to the class that "children with blue eyes are special." At such a young and impressionable age and as one of only two Black children in the class, I took her word for it. It was not until months later when casually repeating this fact to my mom, that I had any inkling that the blue-eyed mythology wasn't true. Let's just say my mother gave that teacher the business! The next day, my teacher apologized and rescinded her statement. But even with an apology, her words had seeped into my psyche and took years to quiet. It wasn't until I read Toni Morrison's *The Bluest Eye* in high school that I began to understand the legacy of consciously work through this psychic wound. When I offer this flower in my workshops and clinical practice, I share it with images of all kinds of babies, as those chocolate cherubs with big brown eyes also evoke the archetypal wisdom of this magical flower. That is why in this text, I refer to the flower as "Baby Eyes."

Baby Eyes addresses a specific type of heartbreak: abandonment and rejection. The original experience of abandonment may have been in our early childhood, or the fear of rejection can develop over time through a series of failed relationships. Relationships that end abruptly without closure or resolution can also result in feelings of abandonment. Abandonment can also be triggered by feeling of being abandoned by God, ancestors, or the spiritual world during exceedingly difficult times.

No matter the source, Baby Eyes is marked by cynicism, a kind that often manifests as cryptic remarks or sarcasm with an underlying expectation that others cannot or will not be responsive to our needs. Baby Eyes also supports us when we armor ourselves against love in an effort to protect ourselves from disappointment or rejection. This becomes a self-fulfilling prophecy: as we protect our hearts from receiving love, we subconsciously push others away until they retreat on their own. We then feel abandoned and rejected all over again! Baby Eyes offers insight and self-awareness to interrupt the self-destructive ride on this merry-go-round.

In the Earth chapter, you'll learn about Mariposa Lily, a flower essence that supports our relationship with the Mother archetype. Baby Eyes is the flower essence that helps us awaken, balance, and heal our relationship with the Father archetype. In the Affirm-a-Flower card deck, Patricia Kaminski offers the affirmation: *My relationship with the Heavenly Father heals my wound with the Earthly Father* by cultivating a relationship with the Divine Masculine in the form of a masculine presence (male or female) who is a provider and source of stability.[58] It is the archetype of the King who offers wise, compassionate leadership and protection. In the Judeo-Christian traditions, Baby Eyes supports our relationship with God, Our Heavenly Father, or Jesus. In African Diasporic traditions, Baby Eyes flower essence aligns us with forces personified with the masculine, such as Obatala and Sango.

As we heal our relationship with the Divine Masculine, our relationships here on Earth also start to shift. I had been estranged from my father for almost twenty years when I began working with Baby Eyes essence. I was in the midst of my own personal transformation and knew that the feelings of abandonment and rejection from childhood were having a negative impact on my dating life. Things would start great, but once physical and emotional intimacy grew, my subconscious fears would kick in and I would project negative expectations onto the relationship. While working with this essence, my father contacted me "out of the blue" through a Facebook message. Much to my own disbelief, I responded and agreed to visit. Baby Eyes opened my willingness to reconcile and helped to cut through years of unprocessed anger, fear, shame, and rejection. It marked the beginning of a new phase in my relationship with my father and an integration of my own masculine that has had a healing effect on all of my relationships.

---

58. *Affirm a Flower Affirmation Deck,* "Baby Blue Eyes" card. Flower Essence Society (FES), www.fesflowers.com.

Embodied Practice: Ustrasana (Camel Pose)

Affirmation: My heart is a portal.

Begin by standing on your knees, with the palms of your hands on your lower back. Gently and with ease, follow your eyes along the ceiling as you gently come into a back bend. As you bend, imagine your hips pressing forward, as your chest opens to the sky. Draw your shoulder blades down and back to deepen the stretch. If you are a beginner, leave your hands on your lower back as you stretch. For a deeper arch, bring one or both hands to your heels, breathing into this deep bend. This pose can be quite intense—only hold it as long as it feels comfortable.

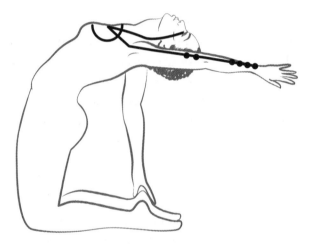

Pictured with the Heart Meridian

Envision a radiant circle of light in your heart. As you inhale, envision light from all four directions expanding this light with warmth and love. As you exhale, envision light radiating from your heart to fill each corner of your room and then the world.

Close your eyes and repeat the affirmation: *My heart is a portal.*

Once complete, slowly and gently draw yourself out of the posture. Come to rest your hips on your heels in a kneeling position. Notice and/or journal any thoughts or feelings that arise.

Soul Lesson 3: Joy Has Juice

Laughter is the sound of the soul dancing.
—Jarod Kintz

Back in the day when I was a cheerleader, one of my favorite cheers went something like this:

"*Smile, Sparkle, Shine it gets 'em every time—*

Smile (clap) Sparkle (clap) Shine!"

The Fire element brings out our ability to sparkle and shine just like the summer sun. (Sidebar: I can't remember where I parked my car, but I still remember the words *and* the movements of this cheer from thirty-plus years ago … go figure!)

As flowers blossom into their unique beauty and glory, our Fire element helps us share our uniqueness with the world. Our hair, our personal style, our posture, and even the sound of our voice can convey to others: I love being me!

Every year, I lead a flower essence excursion in the Brooklyn Botanic Garden to experience different aspects of the garden through the eyes and the ears of the heart. The pavilion with the large border of trees "sounds" authoritative and protective, while the marshy lake "sounds" easygoing and free. We ultimately make our way to the rose sanctuary, which has nearly every species of rose imaginable. Every year, at least one student comments that the rose garden "feels like a party," and I couldn't agree more! As I stroll among the roses, I am aware of an excited exuberance amongst these beauties. The roses are sociable, talkative flowers with lots to say. (By talking, I don't mean that I hear them with my ears—rather, I'm speaking of a way of attuning to a plant's vibe through Alpha and Theta consciousness.) Roses like to laugh and hear stories about good times. They respond to music, humming, and butterflies. They lift the heart with their delight. It's no wonder that roses are one of the quintessential flowers for the Fire element.

Through the Fire element, we learn how to laugh and play with reckless abandon. We learn how to put our responsibilities aside for some plain ol' fun. If you're tired of adulting, it's time to bring in the Fire element. Through Fire, we learn how to include activities, people, and hobbies that bring us joy. Fire invites us to have a sip or two of this "joy juice" every day.

Esteemed scholar and translator of Chinese philosophical texts Elisabeth Rochat de la Vallée explains that the joy of the Fire element has two aspects, *xi* and *le*.[59] Both characters are strongly related to music, and an exploration of these two characters gives us insight into the shamanic origins of Five Element theory. It also helps us to understand the nature of the Fire element today.

The first character, *le*, relates to the music of royal ceremony and ritual.[60] It means "joy, peace, and uplifted spirit."[61] Imagine you are in an ancient temple. The strong pulse of the drums creates a heartbeat, a unified pulse that connects your heart and spirit with the other participants. The music instructs specific rites to be performed at specific time. Today, we can feel this type of unification and joy when we experience African dance. The drum synchronizes the dancers in their representation of cosmic and natural forces through movement. When the drum's rhythm signals the break, *bah dah bop bop, ba dop bop bop!*, the dancers move in sync to the next movement. This shared heartbeat, how we move in sync with others through relationships, is one aspect of the Fire element.

The second character, *xi*, refers to the joy of being in alignment with life, a feeling of internal harmony and excitation. *Xi* is similar to what the French call *joie de vivre*, a natural joy for being alive. This is the kind of internal joy we cultivate through gratitude. We can also turn up this joy with laughter, doing things we love, and enjoying experiences that remind us how good it is to simply be. But what happens when we can't access those feelings of excitement or joy? The Fire element teaches us how to move through the feelings of sadness and isolation so that we can live our best life.

Reflection Questions

Does your joy have juice? Take a moment to reflect on the following questions in your journal:

- What lights up your soul?
- What do you do for fun?
- What makes you laugh out loud?

---

59. Larre, Rochat de la Vallée, and Root, *Seven Emotions*, 106–110.

60. Ibid., 107.

61. Master Wu, 196–212, 204.

+ Who or what sparks your creative passion?
+ When do you most feel vibrant and alive?

Flower Essences for Joy

The following flower essences guide us in awakening our internal joy:

+ California Wild Rose for learning to love life in spite of the thorns
+ Zinnia to laugh out loud
+ Mustard to soak in the sun

California Wild Rose: Love through Thorns—Being happy requires energy. We need California Wild Rose essence when we just don't have the energy to get excited about anything. This flower is helpful when we just don't have any joy juice left to muster up enthusiasm. There is no *joie de vivre*. California Wild Rose also supports us when we're feeling ambivalence or apathy, which can be the result of betrayal, heartache, or extreme stress. Checking out and disengaging from the world is a protective defense mechanism. Sometimes it just hurts too much to care. The problem is that when we numb ourselves to life, we can't experience any joy or love either. As a result, we feel cold, joyless, or indifferent.

I wished California Wild Rose could rain down from the heavens during the spring of 2020. The high school teens I worked with presented profound apathy; saying things such as "it doesn't matter" with accompanying shoulder shrugs. Their hearts had taken a huge hit. Proms, senior trips, graduation ceremonies, and the social rites they looked forward to their whole high school career were indefinitely cancelled due to COVID-19. What was the point in getting excited about anything if it could all just be taken away? This was a classic California Wild Rose moment.

The person needing California Wild Rose may present as vacant, absent, or dulled. There is a sense that the person's inner light (their shen) does not have enough force to actively engage with the world. The person may also complain of feeling disconnected and say things such as, "life is too hard" or "why do I even bother?" California Wild Rose helps us restore our sense of commitment to life or, more accurately, our commitment to being on Earth. This flower essence warms the heart center with the affirmation: *Even though there's heartache, even though there's hardship, I can still engage in life. I don't have to disengage completely to protect myself from pain.* It helps combat the emotional shutdown we experience when turning our hearts off completely so that we don't have to endure any more hurt or pain.

The Fire element reminds us that we are essentially spirit; we are the spark of the divine cosmos that landed in a body. Sometimes we feel as though we didn't sign up for the foolishness of life—the heartache, the disappointment, the highs, and the lows that come with human-beingness. But California Wild Rose helps us accept life's thorns. It is a heart balm that reconnects us to the sweetness of being on Earth.

Zinnia: Laugh Out Loud—Zinnia helps us to awaken the Fire element's capacity for childlike joy, spontaneous adventure, and inhibited exuberance. This flower essence helps us see humor in the curveballs life throws us and encourages us to make time to play. When we take ourselves too seriously, and when we feel overburdened by responsibilities, this cheerful flower whispers in our intuitive ear: "Loosen up! Smile! Relax!"

Zinnia also opens our hearts to experimentation, the play of life, and finding new ways to experience joy. It quiets our inhibitions and our self-critical thoughts, feeling us to try new things. Zinnia also increases spontaneity so that we can step outside the self-imposed limitations and restrictions we put on our lives. While working with Zinnia, I discovered that I could be spontaneous when planned. It sounds oxymoronic, but there was something incredibly healing about allocating small unscheduled chunks of time in my busy life in which I could do whatever brought me joy in that moment. When working with Zinnia, my clients will often receive insight into what they actually enjoy doing that makes them laugh and feel the freedom of the Fire element. Old hobbies and new adventures surface. Zinnia also helps my clients reconnect to the joy embedded in their everyday tasks.

Zinnia flower essence teaches us about reckless abandon, spontaneity, joy, being able to laugh at life, and even being able to laugh at pain. It's a flower recommended for anyone that's lost their joie de vivre, or the connection to the fun and to the whimsy. So this is also a flower essence that I will offer a client who's feeling overwhelmed and overburdened with responsibilities. The Fire element awakens through Zinnia and opens our hearts to more joy, laughter, and fun.

Mustard: Soak in the Sun—In Chinese Medicine, there are five kinds of depression, each related to a specific element. Treatment is not a one-size-fits-all solution but rather based on the specific element and energetics at work.

Water depression comes from weight of sinking qi, which feels as if we can't lift ourselves from the gravitational pull. This type of depression often shows up as fatigue, wanting to sleep, and not getting out of bed. Wood depression shows as an innate feeling of not being able to fulfill our destiny or path. It can be the result of oppression, abuse, or even the sense that for whatever reason, we cannot move upward and forward with ease. Fire's depression feels like someone has blotted out the sun.

Mustard is the flower essence for sadness that sweeps over us like a wave. Sometimes when we experience a crash, it may be followed by the extreme highs and feelings of excitement and mania typical of the Fire element. Mustard provides insight and equanimity to the kind of sadness that descends unexpectedly even and especially when we don't know why. When Mustard is indicated, it's as if we are followed by a cloud of rain, like Eeyore from the children's book, *Winnie the Pooh*. Through this darkness, it is hard to see the good things that are happening all around us.

Listen: depression is nothing to fuck with. The National Institute of Mental Health lists the following symptoms of clinical depression:

+ Persistent sad, anxious, or "empty" mood
+ Feelings of hopelessness or pessimism
+ Feelings of irritability, frustration, or restlessness
+ Feelings of guilt, worthlessness, or helplessness
+ Loss of interest or pleasure in hobbies or activities
+ Decreased energy, fatigue, or being "slowed down"
+ Difficulty concentrating, remembering, or making decisions
+ Difficulty sleeping, early morning awakening, or oversleeping
+ Changes in appetite or unplanned weight changes
+ Aches or pains, headaches, cramps, or digestive problems without a clear physical cause and that do not ease even with treatment
+ Suicide attempts or thoughts of death or suicide[62]

Self-care with flower essences is a great way to support yourself as you move through occasional or passing moods. But if sadness and depression

62. "Depression," National Institute of Mental Health (U.S. Department of Health and Human Services), accessed September 20, 2021, https://www.nimh.nih.gov/health/publications/depression/index.shtml.

persist, please seek help from your medical provider or a health care professional. Do not go it alone. When in doubt, talk it out—with a friend, counselor, spiritual advisor, or therapist.

Embodied Practice: Natarajasana (Dancer Pose)

Affirmation: I dance into joy.

Stand solidly and firmly on your right foot. Bend your left knee, clasping the top of your left foot in your left hand. Either extend your right hand toward the sky, or use a wall to help you find balance. Use your left hand to draw your left foot toward the ceiling. Slowly hinge at the hips. Feel a dynamic tension as you extend your heart, hand, and foot toward the sky, away from one another like an expanding firework.

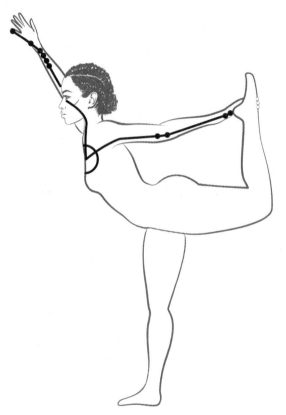

Pictured with the Heart Meridian

Envision that you are a magnet, attracting all the good things in life toward you. Repeat the affirmation: *I dance into joy*.

Repeat on the opposite side.

Soul Lesson 4: Our Senses Are Sacred

Enlightenment is intimacy with all things.
—Dogen Zenji

While all the elements play a role in our sexuality, it is Fire that brings the heat to wield divergent elements into one. Through our sexuality, we can experience the ultimate merging of ourselves into another, a union that can bring us an ecstatic connection with the divine. Many Indigenous practices around the globe include disciplined exercises that cultivate sexual energy for the purpose of sacred union and manifestation.

We start life with the ability to delight in our sensuality. Babies and little children naturally explore their bodies and try to experience the world through all their senses. They put things in their mouth to explore taste and texture. They touch their genitals with reckless abandon. The way the adults respond to this innate sensuality often creates an imprint about how we experience pleasure. The Fire element reveals what has gotten in the way of the natural, organic expression of bodies and sensuality.

Yes, the Fire element is sensual—but sensuality is not felt only in our sexual lives. Western science asks us to use our senses to validate reality. If we cannot taste, touch, see, smell, or hear something, it doesn't exist. The Fire element teaches us that instead of being the gateway between the real and the imagined, our senses are tools to fully and joyously experience the physical world.

As part of my women's leadership program, I teach an intimacy workshop called "Girl 7," inspired by the Spike Lee movie about a sex phone worker. In the workshop, we begin by covering our eyes (hello, blindfolds!) so that we can turn up the volume on our other senses. Each participant is given a sexy substance such as chocolate syrup, honey, marshmallows, ice cream, or whipped cream. (The raunchier workshops include edible lubricants.) I guide the women through an exploration of this sexy substance through the full range of their senses. I invite you to try this sensual mindfulness exercise alone or with a friend.

Practice: Sensual Mindfulness Meditation Script

Begin by covering your eyes. We start by exploring the sensation of touch. Rub the substance on the tips of your fingers to experience its texture and temperature. Is it light and fluffy? Sticky? Dense? Hot or cold? How does it feel as you rub it on your arm or against your cheek? Notice how different parts of your skin are able to experience the sensation of touch.

Next, draw the substance close to you and listen closely to its sound. Does it crackle or whisper? What sounds greet your ear as you shake it, swirl it, stretch it, or squeeze it?

If you are being guided by another person, notice if you try to guess what the substance is, or how quickly you may want to see if you are right. Instead, use this moment to engage your openness and curiosity.

Next we explore scent. Rather than taking a deep inhale, just gently bring this sexy substance close to your nose. Let the scent arrive at the edges of your awareness. Does its aroma draw you closer, or repel you? Is it a sharp scent, or soft and delicate? Our sense of smell is strongly connected to memory. Does its scent remind you of a time, place, or experience? Does your mouth water in anticipation of taste?

Finally, we come to taste. Notice if there is a resonance between the texture and scent as you experience it on the very tip of your tongue. Then, slowly draw the tip of your tongue to the back of your mouth. Does the flavor change as you experience it on your deeper taste buds? Now, bring it completely into your mouth and allow yourself to savor its complexity.

At last, remove your blindfold and gaze as if seeing the substance for the first time. Notice how it is shaped and formed. Describe its variations in color, as well as the way light is reflected or absorbed.

★★★

The goal of the exercise—besides arousal and some fun ideas for the bedroom—is to enjoy an experience with our full being. When we learn to use our senses in this way, life becomes orgasmic. A walk in fresh air, the taste of salty ocean water, the scent from a candle, and the bitterness of dark choc-olate as it melts under our tongue all become invitations to sensuality. We also learn that when we engage our senses in our sex life (and get out of our daggone heads), we experience more emotional intimacy, spiritual connection, and physical orgasm.

I call on the Fire element whenever someone is having a hard time in their sexual relationships, especially if they are uncomfortable talking about sex, masturbation, or pleasure. The Fire element supports us when we need to access sources of personal pleasure, sensuality, and ecstasy outside of our actual sex life. So yes, we want great sex with great orgasms, and nature has our back. But we also need experiences of ecstasy, joy, and pleasure in our everyday life. The Fire element teaches us how to welcome an ecstatic connec-tion to life on Earth.

Reflection Questions

Do you experience your senses as sacred? Take a moment to reflect on the following questions in your journal:

+ What role does sensuality play in your life?
+ What flavors, aromas, sounds, and textures do you most enjoy?
+ How is your sensuality expressed?
+ In which relationships do you experience emotional intimacy, sexual intimacy, or both?
+ Are there any wounds that inhibit your sexual expression?
+ What brings you pleasure? What brings you joy?

Flower Essences for Our Sacred Senses

The following flower essences for the Fire element help us access our sensual nature and support us as we explore the blocks that get in the way:

+ Hibiscus for emotional and sexual intimacy
+ Pretty Face for inner and outer beauty
+ Pussy Paws for titillating touch

Hibiscus: Emotional and Sexual Intimacy—At the risk of making the others jealous, Hibiscus is hands down one of my favorite flower essences. Developing a relationship with and expertise about one flower is a requirement for flower essence practitioner certification. When it was time for me to take on this massive research project, Hibiscus showed up for me again and again.

Before I talk about Hibiscus, let me tell you the tale of Swaggalicious. What is a Swaggalicious, you ask? Well. A Swaggalicious is a person—male, female, or nonbinary—who has so much daggone swag that all you want to do is have sex. May you be so blessed to find this person at least once in your life. Maybe it's the size and shape of their physique that turns you on, but usually it's something else—the way they smile, walk, move in their bodies, their voice, their personal style. Whatever it is, part of you melts when you are around them. And though it *can* happen in theory, a Swaggalicious doesn't typically turn into a lasting relationship. They are messy. Sometimes emotionally unavailable. Sometimes married. Sometimes, just a whole hot mess on every level. I thought I was the only one with a Swaggalicious, but the more I talk to my friends and clients, the more I know that there are many out there roaming the earth and igniting fires with all that swag.

One of my clients kept her Swaggalicious on deck for over five years, even though she knew he did not want a long-term, monogamous relationship with her. Every few months they would meet to have fantastic sex in an exotic location. Over time, they would stay at each other's houses, even starting to crack the layers. And without fail, after these moments of emotional intimacy, he would either disappear or my client would stop taking his calls.

You may be wondering what Swaggalicious has to do with Hibiscus. Hibiscus flower essence helps to explore our relationship between emotional and sexual intimacy. Some of us use our sexuality to deepen emotional connection. Some of us use sex to create emotional distance. Some of us withhold sex to create emotional distance, while some of us withhold sex to create space for emotional connection. See how quickly this gets confusing? And some of us do all of the above, depending on the relationship. Hibiscus flower essence helps give insight into the blocks that keep our emotional and sexual intimacy from living together harmoniously in one relationship.

Working with Hibiscus as one of her key flowers, my client began to explore the moments she welcomed Swaggalicious into her bed. We discovered that she called him whenever a new relationship gained some traction. Swaggalicious was there to keep her from getting too close to her potential partner, by dissipating some of the intensity of her fear. She also called Swaggalicious to reset when ending relationships. If she knew she wanted to break up with someone but didn't have the words or the nerve? Yup, you guessed it. She called her Swaggalicious.

Hibiscus flower essence facilitates a beautiful connection between the heart and the sexual energetic centers, especially when the two have been estranged. The flower is an adaptogen, meaning that it can be either warming or cooling, depending on what we need. It balances Fire and Water: if your sexual energy or heart feels cold or dry, Hibiscus will warm, lubricate, and get things flowing. (This is why the flower essence is often indicated for menopausal women.) When sexual forces are too fired up, Hibiscus cools the fires enough to invite our heart into the mix. Either way, Hibiscus helps us to integrate sexual and emotional intimacy so that we can experience both in a balanced, authentic way.

In her essay, *The Erotic as Power*, prolific writer Audre Lorde explores the role of sensuality in consciousness. She critiques how our society comes to understand the feminine body as an object. My good friend Deneen translated this article for me by explaining that too often, women's bodies are basically "sexual furniture." In advertisements, music videos, radio songs, YouTube videos, and social media, we often see images of our bodies as something to be observed or displayed, but devoid of feeling and sensation. At the same time, we are often exposed to the fetishization of certain bodies through the media's patriarchal male gaze. The numbness in our bodies may reflect our armoring and desensitization to shield us from explicit sexual images or language.

Our sensuality is meant to be embodied. Whether we identify as male, female, or non-binary, Hibiscus revitalizes our sensitivity to the vital force of eros flowing through our veins. Hibiscus invites us to ask ourselves: How is my sexual expression an expression of love, and how is my love reflected in my sexual expression? The flower essence guides us as we explore any blocks in our physical, emotional, and sexual expression. Are we able to bring our sexuality into relationships as an extension of our love—including self-love? Hibiscus helps us explore the relationship we have with our own sensual selves and address any wounding of our sexual expression. Hibiscus reminds us that sexuality, passion, sensitivity, and love are intimately connected.

Pretty Face: Inner and Outer Beauty—When you look in the mirror, what do you see? Do you give yourself positive affirmations about the things you love? Or do you fixate on what you don't like about yourself? Pretty face (*Triteleia ixioides*) evokes the inner African goddess Osun, who is often depicted gazing at her reflection in the mirror. It is a flower essence that addresses both sides of the polarity of vanity—it is possible to be too vain, and it is also problematic if we are not vain enough. Pretty Face teaches us that pretty is as pretty does and helps us see, appreciate, and radiate our personal beauty in the world.

We live in a society where pretty privilege is real. Attractive people tend to be more social, get better discounts, and skip long lines. But the current standard of beauty is full of fuckery. Western culture has a pretty narrow definition of beauty: white, thin, young, and able-bodied. I don't know the exact numbers, but in my imaginings, this definition excludes something like 90 percent of the people on the planet. This is especially heightened now in the age of social media, where we take an alarming number of selfies and where our images live in cyberspace *forever*. There has arguably never been more pressure to be beautiful.

Pretty Face helps us explore socially imposed standards of beauty and how these standards consciously or unconsciously affect us. I often share this flower's wisdom with my high school girls. Unfortunately, the amount of colorism and anti-Black messages that pervade pop culture don't seem to be shifting fast enough. My mother grew up in the rural south in the 1950s, where Black skin needed to be lighter than a brown paper bag to be considered beautiful. Fast-forward seventy years, and my daughter listens to songs on the radio where being yellow-boned (translation: light complexion) is a requirement for sexiness. I cringed in season 1 of the sitcom *Community*, when the blond-haired protagonist innocently suggests that biracial couples make the cutest children. I mean, come on. Seriously?!?!?

As woke and evolved as we claim to be, our society has a *lot* of work to do with Pretty Face. (And quite honestly, with anti-racism in general. But we'll leave that quest to the Wood element). Author and activist Sonya Renee Taylor brings the negative, socially imposed views about our bodies into sharp focus in her book, *The Body Is Not an Apology: The Power of Radical Self-Love*.[63] In it, she explores the origins of guilt and shame we may feel when we

---

63. Sonya Renee Taylor, *The Body Is Not an Apology: The Power of Radical Self-Love* (Oakland, CA: Berrett-Koehler Publishers, 2018).

look in the mirror, as well as action steps to change the nature of the relationships we have with ourselves through radical care. She writes:

> Our earliest memories of body shame left us with a sense that something was wrong with us, that our bodies should be different than they were (while consequently being the same as the other bodies around us). How we decided what our bodies should look like was formed in part by the messages we received. Those messages were transmitted and reinforced by culture, society, politics, and our families. Those messages stuck with us.[64]

Pretty Face ushers in a deep respect for the body in all shapes and forms, colors, and contexts. When we look in the mirror and focus on our flaws, Pretty Face chides us with a loving "Hush all that nonsense! You are beautiful as you are, your body is exactly as it needs to be." It is an ally for anyone questioning their attractiveness. It's also a flower essence that I recommend—with appropriate therapy and counseling—for dysmorphia, a condition in which a person has a skewed perspective of their body with obsessive attention given to their perceived imperfections. What they see in the mirror is not what others see. Pretty Face helps us to be "flawsome" and accept what we perceive as imperfections as part of our whole, divine package.

The Fire element teaches us how to get naked, physically and emotionally. What we see in the mirror and how we internalize what others see are real things. But our relationship with our own body is sacred and intimate. I learned this Pretty Face lesson through my work with photographer Sparkle Davian. During her boudoir photo parties, she would mist Pretty Face in the air to support the confidence of her clients. When preparing for my own boudoir shoot, she calmed my nerves by explaining:

> I'm not going to ask about your outfits. What's more important is, how do you feel? I want women to know that the sexiest piece of lingerie is not a leather corset, a G-string thong, or a push-up bra…it is and will always be confidence. If a woman embraces the concept

64. Taylor, *The Body Is Not an Apology*, 34.

that *every* woman has a beauty all her own, it will radiate through her eyes, her posture, and the simple peek of her shoulder.[65]

Pretty Face teaches how to—in true Osun fashion—adorn ourselves! It helps us to see the things that we like about ourselves and play them up a bit. This flower essence guides you as you learn how to appreciate and draw attention to your favorite parts (and away from your not-so-favorite parts). I personally love my eyes and my breasts, so you'll find me in glittery eye shadows and v-neck tops. Do you love your hands? Embellish them with unique rings and bracelets. Love your smile? Try a new bright or glittery lip gloss. Love to stand out? Rock some bright and bold colors. I see you, Pretty Face, in my bruthas with their sexy groomed beards and fresh kicks. It doesn't matter our gender; Pretty Face invites us to find the things we love about ourselves and to show them off to the world. The important lesson this flower teaches is how to see your beauty—inside and out—and how to love it fiercely.

In spite of (or perhaps because of) the messages she received as a child, my mom is the reigning pretty face champion. When I visited her in the hospital after her cancer surgery, she had already managed to have the nurses apply a bright, bold red lipstick. She has closets full of shoes, jewelry, and beautiful things she uses to celebrate and adorn herself. I've never seen her not look fabulous. Even during COVID, my mom would show up to Zoom calls with a fully done face, fly outfit, and matching jewelry. Pretty Face would be proud. That's how you do it folks!

Pussy Paws: Titillating Touch—I spent my twentieth birthday doing a study abroad in Paris. I can effortlessly relive the sights, sounds, and smells of this beautiful city. I fondly remember my mornings on the balcony with my coffee and breakfast baguette drizzled with honey, trying hard not to hear my host family having loud, passionate sex a few rooms over. Paris is indeed a sexy city.

While I was there, I made a several life-changing friendships: a fashion photographer who introduced me to the underground hip hop scene, the Black American woman I babysat for, and an unlikely friendship with Claire, a fifty-year old white woman with a spirit for adventure. One evening she took me to her friends' house for a gathering, with the most delicious food on

---

65. Sparkle Davian (boudoir photographer) in conversation with the author, March 2019.

planet Earth. Her friends called me *gourmand*. I didn't know what it meant, so I consulted my pocket French-English dictionary (yes, this was before smartphones and Google). The dictionary said that *gourmand* meant "greedy." I felt immediately self-conscious and insulted.

I asked Claire why her friends were so rude as to call me greedy—and to my face! Was it because they thought I didn't understand the language (which was partially true)? Claire laughed and explained to me that being called *gourmand* is a compliment in French and a word that doesn't have an English equivalent. It meant something along the lines of having a fine appreciation for delicious things, sharing the same root as the word "gourmet." It means delighting in the textures, tastes, and aromas of cuisine. In other words, I was a "foodie."

I think of that story whenever I think of Pussy Paws flower essence. The flower looks so much like a little, fluffy cotton ball that it makes you want to rub it on your cheek. Pussy Paws flower essence awakens us to the deliciousness of touch, one of the five senses that we often take for granted. The delight that a foodie feels when having an exquisite gourmet meal is the same rapture that Pussy Paws helps us awaken as we experience the textures of the world.

Invariably on dating apps, someone will ask, "What's your love language?" I've seen some *very* creative (and concerning) answers to this question! But the discussion prompt refers to a book by Gary Chapman, called the *Five Love Languages: How to Express Heartfelt Commitment to Your Mate*.[66] The book has gained so much traction and popularity that there have been a number of spinoffs: *The Five Love Languages of Children*, *The Five Love Languages of Teens*, *The Five Love Languages for Educators*, and so on. Part of what makes the concepts so applicable across the wide span of relationships is that the desire to love and be loved is deeply encoded in the human psyche. I relate Chapman's archetypal love patterns to the five elements:

1. Quality Time: Water—meaningful experiences that create trust and connection over time
2. Words of Affirmation: Wood—using our words to compliment, affirm, and celebrate one another

66. Gary D. Chapman and Amy Summers, *The Five Love Languages: How to Express Heartfelt Commitment to Your Mate* (Nashville, TN: LifeWay Press, 2010).

3. Acts of Service: Earth—offering energy or time with consideration of how to make someone's life easier

4. Gifts: Metal—offering a symbol from the material world to represent something spiritual or intangible (including love)

5. Physical Touch: Fire—connection and intimacy through touch

Let's talk for a moment about this physical touch piece. Remember, the Fire element is involved with any and every relationship, no matter the style of expression But the Fire element is especially turned on (or off) by the nature of intimate touch and affection.

Pussy Paws teaches how to incorporate safe, appropriate, and loving touch into our relationships. The key word here is *appropriate*. It's not appropriate to, as Donald Trump was recoded saying, "grab 'em by the pussy." Violent physical touch (and language) reverberates through our nervous system, shocks the heart, and scatters the shen. Our Fire element also responds to touch that lacks clarity or integrity. That hug or comment from a colleague that leaves us asking, "What the fuck was that?" will alert our spidey senses. Pussy Paws will bring into our conscious awareness the experiences of touch that we have not yet reconciled.

Pussy Paws also supports us if we have an aversion to touch. This could range from a startled jump when someone touches you to full-on *Matrix*-style backbends to resist a hug. Physical intimacy, or lack thereof, can make or break the most loving relationships, and this flower essence can be a powerful ally for couples who struggle with their sexual connection. Finding new ways to connect through touch, such as massage, hugs, or holding hands, can open the doors for intimacy in even the most challenged relationships. The flower essence helps us to explore the underlying reason for physical aversion, and to move through it so that it does not become a block to emotional intimacy.

Pussy Paws will also expand our awareness of how to create appropriate touch in nonsexual relationships. For example, the teenager who is exploring their own body may not be as into hugs as they used to be. But if physical touch is their love language, they may crave tactile affirmation of care. Stuffed animals, cool fabrics, or a handshake may fill that void. At home or in the workplace where you intuit the need for physical touch, try a high five, fist bump, or a pound instead of going in for the hug. I love those videos of teachers who create a special handshake for each kid in the class; it's a powerful example of the Fire element in action.

Pause for a moment to rub your fingertips together. Notice the sensations between your fingertips. Draw your fingers along the edges of your arms. Touch your clothes, and sense the shape of your body beneath the layers. Pussy Paws supports this attention to texture and touch. Of course, this is beneficial in sexual intimacy, where our experience of touch is extremely important. This includes the sensations on our fingertips, the sensations along the vaginal walls or on the shaft of the penis, the sensations on our erogenous zones, or the even the sensations on the places on our bodies we don't pay attention to. Pussy Paws awakens the skin's sensitivity. I've had students share that when they're taking pussy paws flower essence, even the simple act of putting on shea butter in the morning becomes a sensual experience.

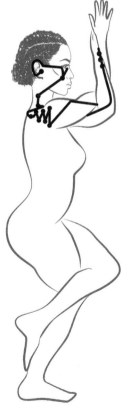

Embodied Practice: Garudasana(Eagle Pose)

Affirmation: My senses are sacred.

Stand firmly on your right foot, rooting into the ground. Slowly raise your left knee, crossing it over your right as you sink into a gentle squat. Once you find your balance, swoop your left arm beneath your right, crossing at the elbows and again at your wrists to clasp the palms of your hands together. (If this feels uncomfortable, rest your hands on your shoulders in the self-hug position.)

Your perineum muscles are the muscles you would use to stop your pee midstream. Squeeze and release your perineum muscles three times to create a pulsing sensation.

Bring your attention to places your skin touches.

Close your eyes and rest as you repeat the affirmation: *My senses are sacred.* Repeat on the opposite side.

Pictured with the Small Intestine Meridian

Music Is Medicine: Playlist for the Fire Element

Fire element songs awaken your sensuality, and activate your heart forces. Though every love song belongs to the Fire element, the songs on this list evoke additional signatures and sounds of Fire. These songs remind us not only about romantic love but also the Fire element's love for life and the spark of divinity we share.

"Best Day of My Life" by American Authors
Album: Oh, What a Lie, *Mercury-Island, 2013*

My best friend and I play this song whenever we are in a bad mood. It's such a happy song, filled with the life and liveliness of the Fire element. The Fire element teaches us how to embrace each day with exuberance and joy. When we wake and greet the day screaming, "this is the best day of my life," we are activating Fire's excited celebration.

"Turn Down for What?" by DJ Snake and Lil Jon
Single, Columbia Records, 2013

I double dog dare you to sit still while this song is playing. The Fire element is the most yang of all the elements. The energy of this song brings us up and out, ready to move and turn up. It sounds like a fuse that is about to explode! And once we're up experiencing the highs of the Fire element, who the heck wants to come down?

"Mood 4 Eva" by Beyoncé, Jay-Z and Childish Gambino
Album: The Lion King: The Gift, *Parkwood Columbia, 2019*

Speaking of enjoying ourselves, "Mood 4 Eva" taps into the joy and celebration of the Fire element when we reach the heights of success. This song was written for the 2019 live action adaptation of *The Lion King,* and its melody was inspired by the classic "Hakuna Matata" no worries vibe. The Fire element teaches us how to put our cares aside and live our lives like it's a great big party.

"Dance Tonight" by Lucy Pearl
Album: Lucy Pearl, *Virgin Records, 2000*

The Fire element is with us whenever we're dancing, celebrating, and feeling free. Even that Amazon binge shopping spree is calling in a taste of the Fire element. Fire reminds us that life is meant to be enjoyed—and we should look and feel good doing it. Fire screams, "Look at me shine!" Whether you pop bottles or pop your collar, that's Fire.

"La Vie en Rose" by Grace Jones,
Album: Portfolio, *Island Records, 1977*

This song was originally written and performed by Edith Piaf in 1943 but has since then been covered a bazillion times. My favorite rendition is by goddess Grace Jones. "La Vie en Rose" tells the story of a young woman who has fallen madly in love. Her world has a rosy tint to it, making even the hardest times feel light and free. When we are madly in love with life, we are kissed and blessed by the Fire element. Fire helps us see the world through rose-colored glasses—with optimism and joy.

"You're Never Fully Dressed Without a Smile" by Sia
Album: Annie, *Columbia-Roc Nation Records, 2014*

Fire element is classically diagnosed through a laughing voice. This voice sounds like it's smiling, even when it's upset. The song brings us back to the childlike wonder of the movie *Annie,* which I grew up on and was remixed for a new generation in 2014. The song is delightful. With Fire, we evoke a child-like energy. This song reminds us that smiling (and laughing) is a surefire way to activate our Fire element qi.

"Eternal Flame" by the Bangles
Album: Everything, *CBS/Liberation, 1989*

The lead singer of this song has a classic Fire element voice. If you close your eyes, you can almost imagine her smiling behind lyrics that convey her deep longing. The Fire element lights our hearts with passion and desire, and this song reminds us that love is eternal.

"Skin" by Rihanna
Album: Loud, Def Jam Recordings, 2010

This song is super sexy, as are all things by the siren Rihanna. In "Skin," we feel the smoldering sensuality of the Fire element. Fire teaches us how to embrace, enjoy, and delight in the pleasure of touch. It awakens us to the textures and sensations that our skin encounters. The Fire element teaches us all about pleasure—not just the pleasure of sex, but pleasure as the foundation of our being.

"Naked" by Ella Mai
Album: Ella Mai, 10 Summers/Interscope, 2018

My friend and colleague teaches a series of yoga workshops based on the principle of "bringing sacredness to nakedness."[67] Though some people balk at the idea of practicing yoga completely nude, The Naked Yoga Goddess reminds us of a lesson at the heart of the Fire element: we want nothing more than to be seen as we are and loved fully. Like Fire, this song and my friend teach us that being naked is not just about being bare physically—it's also about the vulnerability we feel when we are emotionally exposed. The Fire element drives our desire to be loved despite our flaws and insecurities and melts the wall of ice we build to hide and protect our heart.

"Pressure" by Ari Lennox
Single, Dreamville/Interscope, 2021

This flirty, sultry songstress captures the playful essence of the Fire element in "Pressure." The Fire element helps us to release our inhibitions and have the confidence to ask for what brings us joy and pleasure. Whether we are in the bedroom or in the boardroom, the Fire element is there to make sure that we are living our most orgasmic life.

---

67. Kimberly Baker Simms, TheNakedYogaGoddess.com, in conversation with the author, February 2021.

"A Rose Is Still a Rose" by Aretha Franklin
Album: A Rose Is Still A Rose, *Arista Records, 1998*

The rose is the quintessential flower of the Fire element, and has been a heart healer since the ancient world. This song reminds us of the perseverance and resilience of the heart. A rose is exquisitely beautiful—just like our lives—even though it has its thorns. The Fire element reminds us that no matter what bumps and bruises we encounter along the way, the heart remains as pure and beautiful as a rose.

"Como la Flor" by Selena
Album: Entre En Mi Mundo, *EMI Latin, 1992*

The joyous, dancing melody of "Como La Flor" resonates with the Fire element. In the lyrics, songbird Selena compares her heart to a romantic flower that was given to a lover. In the Fire phase of any romance, love blossoms abundantly. But every season changes, and just like a flower, without Fire's affection and attention, the love in her heart ultimately wilts and dies.

"Love thy Will be Done" by Martika
Album: Martika's Kitchen, *Sony Music, 1991*

Many people overlook this B-side track written by the artist formerly known as Prince and performed by Martika. "Love thy Will be Done" connects us to the majestic divinity of the Fire element, reminding us of the sacredness of a life unfolding as it should. This song directs the love in our hearts to the exquisite perfection of a higher power. The Fire element teaches us how to love life and all creation as through the eyes of the Divine, no matter what we experience as mere mortals.

Fire in Practice: Make Time for Joy

The Fire element inspires us to live a life full of joy, intimacy, play, excitement, connection, and passion. The problem is that sometimes we get so wrapped up in our daily grind, we forget to make time for the people, places, or experiences that feed our soul. Use the guidelines below to generate a list of activities that tend the flames of your Fire element.

Illuminations

When it gets dark, it's time to turn on the lights! The activities on our *Illuminations* list should be easy and accessible without taking a lot of time, money, or effort. Our *Illuminations* keep the light in our hearts steady and resilient. We can aim to do at least one of these practices every day.

Examples:

+ Listening to music or a favorite playlist
+ Cooking favorite foods
+ Morning coffee (the bitter taste of coffee is associated with the Fire element!)
+ Taking a bubble bath or a luxuriously long shower
+ Using a fave perfume, soap, or body product
+ Chatting with a friend
+ Cuddling with a loved one
+ Spending time in nature
+ Playing with pets
+ Puzzles or coloring books
+ Prayer
+ Meditation
+ Exercise (easy and manageable, like a fifteen-minute yoga class or walk)
+ Reading a book you enjoy
+ Working on a passion project

Candles

The next set of activities to identify are your *Candles*. Like candles, the activities on this list are lit periodically or ritualistically to make sure our Fire element has a healthy glow. Plan to light these candles regularly—weekly or even monthly—as they require more effort and planning than daily *Illuminations*.

Examples:

+ Attending a class or workshop in a topic that you are passionate about
+ Going out to dinner or to the movies
+ Playing on a sports team

- Buying or picking fresh flowers
- Family or friends game night
- Leisurely shopping
- Dance or exercise class
- Creative solitude (including fasts from social media)
- Getting dressed up
- Experimenting with a new or gourmet recipe
- Taking a day trip to a local attraction (museums, garden, comedy club, beach, etc.—check for your city's local listings of free events and activities)
- Full moon/New moon rituals
- Visiting family that lives a further distance
- Date night (with yourself or a partner)
- Massage or acupuncture treatment
- Watching (or binge-watching) a favorite show
- Sex or physical intimacy (depending on your libido, this might be worked into your daily routine)

Fireworks

Fireworks are reserved for special occasions and celebrations. We participate in the activities on our *Fireworks* list less frequently because they may require significant planning, time, or financial commitment. They have the potential to reset our pilot light, jumpstart our heart, and relieve stress. We can plan our *Fireworks* seasonally, annually, or those special moments when our Fire element needs a boost.

Examples:

- Spa day
- Vacation/travel
- Wine festival
- Concert
- Amusement park
- Photo shoot
- Get a make-over (change your hairstyle, revamp your wardrobe, etc.)
- Throw a party
- Outdoor adventures (skiing, hiking, camping, rock climbing, etc.)

- Hot-air balloon ride
- Water activities (boating, sailing, kayaking, windsurfing, jet skiing, etc.)
- Spiritual initiation or rites

Once you've generated your lists, it's time to pull out your personal calendar! See if you can allocate time for the activities you've identified, including practices from each category. Be sure to offer gratitude for the privilege and blessing of being able to celebrate your light!

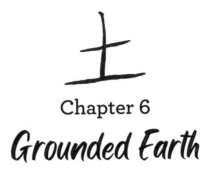

Chapter 6

Grounded Earth

The Earth element phase ripens after Fire element. When the Earth element is grounded and balanced, we nurture the needs of our bodies, our family, and our community. We make dietary and health choices in service of physical, emotional, and spiritual health. Just as we are nourished by food, the Earth element helps us digest our experiences. Our actions give substance to brilliance that we are ready to manifest.

Earth Element Signatures

We can recognize the archetypal qualities of the Earth element through the following signatures:

- Season: Late summer; transitions between seasons
- Phase: Fruit
- Color: Yellow
- Energetic: Spins qi
- Core Emotions: Empathy, resonance
- Sound: Singing
- Meridians: Stomach and Spleen

Season: Late Summer

In some acupuncture texts, the Earth element is associated with late summer, a time when the air becomes heavy and sticky with humidity. The sluggishness and the lethargy we experience on a hot, sticky day is very resonant with the experience of an imbalanced Earth element. However, in the cosmological sequence of the five elements, Earth holds the axis position of a wheel that places Fire in the south, Water in the north, Wood in the east, and Metal in the west:

> When the Earth is placed in the centre, its role in relation to the seasons is apparent. The Earth actually belongs to no season as it is the neutral pivot along which the seasonal cycle unfolds... The Earth does perform the role of replenishment at the end of each season. Thus at the end of each season, the energy goes back to the Earth for regeneration.[68]

The Earth element brings a stabilizing energy that helps us to anchor in the midst of change. In my clinical practice, I call on the Earth element to help a person stay centered and embodied while the world shifts around them. The Earth element is associated with our home, environment, physical body, and connection to nature. Our relationship to our earthly mother, pregnancy, and fertility are all within its domain.

This element also supports us as we accumulate, digest, and assimilate emotions and our experiences, in addition to how our soul is nourished by all that we consume. Study and mental processes that require focus and the integration of large quantities of information rely on the Earth element for success. Because this element is of substance, Earth supports the art of manifestation and our ability to bring abstract thoughts and ideas out of the ethers and into the material world.

Phase: Fruit

In the life cycle of nature, the flower is followed by the fruit. The Earth element calls to mind the cornucopia of abundance, overflowing in its ability to nourish and sustain life. When we celebrate the fruits of our labor, we are taking a moment to acknowledge the gifts and blessings that we experience as a reward for our commitment and dedication.

Similarly, in our life cycle as we blossom and fill with abundance and love, we are compelled to offer ourselves in service to others. The Earth element supports our capacity to offer emotional, physical, or spiritual nourishment to ourselves and those we care for. It is associated with the archetypal Mother

---

68. Giovanni Maciocia, *The Foundations of Chinese Medicine* (Edinburgh, UK: Elsevier Churchill Livingstone, 2005), 30.

and how we bring love and care into the world, just as Mother Earth sustains and nurtures all life on the planet.

Color: Yellow

The color of the Earth element is golden yellow, like the bright color of sunflowers, dandelions, and fields of wheat. We find gold in the vibrant leaves as they change colors in the fall. Corn, which has a long association in Native American culture with the cycles and rhythms of Mother Earth, reflects the Earth element's golden signature.

Energetic: Spins Qi

Just as Earth rotates on its axis, the energetic movement of the Earth element is circular and winding. The round quality of the Earth element evokes the symbol of the community circle. Rather than hierarchical relationships where one person is better or higher in the ranks, Earth emphasizes relationships where we all come together as equals for the common good. The spinning of the planet also creates the gravitational pull. In the same way, healthy Earth element qi helps us to feel centered, grounded, and solidly in our bodies.

The circular, winding movement of qi is also referred to as overthinking. When out of balance, the Earth element will spin our thoughts around and around such that they never resolve or materialize. This circular thought pattern can be experienced as anxiety or worry. It shows up when we're thinking about something over and over again, but we can't figure out how to either make it happen or make it better.

Core Emotion: Empathy, Resonance

The Earth element gifts us with the capacity to have compassion for the suffering of others, as well as to share the joys of humanity. We experience sympathetic resonance whenever we casually say to a friend, "I feel you." This expresses the Earth's compassion, because we are essentially saying, "I get you.

I understand you. I share this human experience with you." The Earth element teaches us sympathy and empathy; and how to lend our support, kindness, concern, and care. When in balance, we're able to feel into each other's needs. We read and respond to nonverbal cues and can respond appropriately. When out of balance, we may lack the emotional sensitivity required for healthy relationships. In other case, imbalanced Earth causes us to take on too much of the environment or other people's feelings, such that we lose our energetic center. The Earth element helps to bring us back to ourselves so that we can be calm, grounded, and clear. Additional emotions and sensations associated with the Earth element include:

Worry	Anxiety	Dysmorphia
Grounded	Centered	Empathy
Sympathy	Overthinking	Stangnation
Lethargy	Unclear	Confusion
Heaviness	Ungrounded	Mental Fuzziness

The Earth element aligns closely with the etheric layer of the subtle body (sometimes called the emotional or energetic body). Even if the phrase is new to you, we've all experienced some aspect of the etheric body. Have you ever felt as though someone was staring at you and when you turn around, someone has you in their steady gaze? They are not touching you physically, they are touching you energetically. Because our emotions live mostly in our etheric body, etherically sensitive folks tend to be very empathic and can often sense when someone is feeling angry or sad, even if their words indicate otherwise. Being in crowds can upset the nervous system of etherically sensitive folks, who might need to spend some time decompressing alone after lots of interaction with others.

Not only are we connected to each other, we are also connected to the earth herself. The Schumann Resonance refers to the electromagnetic energies that are responsible for the changing seasons, tides, and weather patterns. If you feel a little more emotional during a full moon, that reflects your connection to the Schumann Resonance. Our electromagnetic bodies are in close synergy with the electromagnetic poles of Earth, and etherically sensitive folks are often affected by eclipses, equinoxes, solstices, and changes in the weather. If your back hurts 'cuz it's cold outside, you gain a few extra pounds during your monthly cycle, or your knee acts up every time it rains, you know exactly what I mean. The feelings of connection and solace we experience when we spend time in nature are also an extension of this resonance. Folk wisdom and spiritual medicine are deeply rooted in our relationship with the rhythms, seasons, and energies of the earth.

Sound: Singing

The sound of the Earth element in a person's voice is "singing," with melodic highs and lows that resemble a soothing lullaby. We can hear the Earth element in our voices by imagining we are asking a toddler, "oooooh, do you have a boo boo?" We can hear the Earth element in songs that have a soothing, melodic quality. Music that conveys a sense of "roundness," and lyrics that expresses neediness, solidarity, or compassion also resonate strongly with the Earth element. We also hear the Earth element in songs that affirm our interdependence and the bonds that connect us as a family, tribe, nation, or human race.

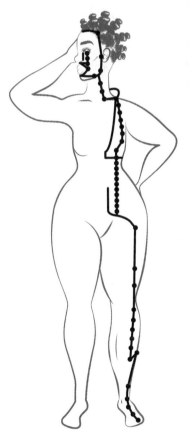

6.1 Stomach Meridian

Meridians: Spleen and Stomach

The Spleen and Stomach are the internal organs associated with the Earth element, which is in charge of our digestion. This is not only how we digest our food but also includes our ability to digest information, emotions, and experiences. The health of our Earth element determines how well we are nourished by our life.

The Stomach meridian [**Figure 6.1**] starts just beneath the eye, descends along the cheek and jaw before ascending to the top of the head. From there, it travels down the front of the body, the front of the thigh and shin, and the top of the foot before ending at the tip of the fourth toe. The Spleen meridian [**Figure 6.2**] starts in the inside corner of the big toe, travels along the inside of the footbefore climbing along the inner leg and thigh. Near the groin, the meridian dives into the abdominal cavity, then emerges along the lateral side of the chest before ending on the side of the ribcage. When the Earth element is imbalanced, we may experience some of the following symptoms:

+ Digestive issues
+ Weight gain
+ Weak muscles
+ Emotional eating
+ Blood disorders
+ Headaches/head fogginess
+ Fatigue/lethargy, especially after eating
+ Mucus or phlegm
+ Sugar cravings

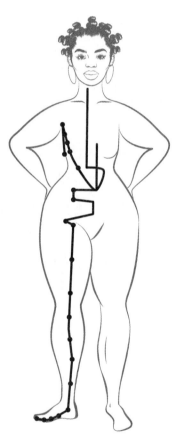

The Earth element benefits from a healthy diet that avoids excesses. Earth is nourished by mindful eating and a diet that includes a variety of fruits, vegetables, grains, and proteins eaten at regular intervals. In yoga, poses which strengthen the digestive fire in the solar plexus and those with twists and binds activate Earth, while balancing postures allow us to experience Earth's stability under our feet. The Earth element meridians run along the shins and front of the thighs; gentle massage on these areas will also nourish the Earth element. Finally, the Earth element can be evoked

6.2 Spleen Meridian

in any yoga practice that incorporates loving self-care and acknowledges the physical body's magnificence as a temple for the spirit.

Soul Lesson 1: Honor the Mothers

Be wildly devoted to devoted to someone, or something.
Cherish every perception.
At the same time, forget about control.
Allow the Beloved to be herself, and to change.
—*The Radiance Sutras*, Verse 98

The Latin root of our word "material," *mater*, means mother. No matter how you slice and dice it, everything in the physical, manifested universe was born through a mother. The Mother archetype has existed since the beginning of life itself. One of my teachers, Baba Ifasanmi Adesanya Awoyade, frequently reminds his godchildren that, "if you have a belly button, you have a mother." Through the Earth element, we are called to honor not only our birth mother, but the collective mothers who nurture all life—cosmic mothers, spiritual mothers, our caretakers (male or female), and Mother Earth itself. Everything we experience in our earthly existence is because the divine mothers of creation have allowed it to materialize. Whenever I want to manifest something important—a new project, a partner, financial abundance, or spiritual growth—I imagine these mothers smiling down on me. "Mother, may I?"

Yes, you may.

The mother principle creates and nurtures the physical vessel for spirit to come into existence in the material world. Additional archetypes associated with the Mother include the Caregiver, the Nurturer, the Teacher, the Rescuer, and the Healer. The Earth element supports us in activating these archetypes with in our psyche. In *The Hero and the Outlaw*, authors divide twelve contemporary consumer-culture archetypes into four primal needs of the human psyche. The Nurturer/Caregiver archetype is categorized with the archetypes that serve to provide structure to the world.[69] It is midway between

---

69. Margaret Mark and Carol S. Pearson, *The Hero and the Outlaw: Harnessing the Power of Archetypes to Create a Winning Brand* (New York: McGraw-Hill, 2002), 205–262.

the Ruler and the Creator archetypes in the same category. This force of the psyche is responsible for giving form to the invisible.

Our existence begins as a thought, recognized or unrecognized, in our parents' minds. Once conceived, we are nestled in our mama's womb for nine months, receiving the nutrients we need to become bones, blood, flesh, mind, and soul. There are many things that could go wrong along the course of this intricate process. Depending on our unique circumstances, conditions were either optimal or not. But if you are reading (or listening to) this book, enough went right that you were born into the world. The Earth element supports the miraculous process through which something goes from being an idea—pure spirit—into a manifested entity in the physical world.

The Earth element governs this path of embodiment. This process is at work on macro and micro levels whenever we are birthing something, whether it be a baby, a business, or a book. The Earth element helps us take our vision and ideas to make them tangible, practical, and earthbound. This is how we manifest the life we want. But just like a baby in a womb, manifestation doesn't happen overnight. It requires dedication, commitment, devotion, and daily nurturance. This is the humble work of the Earth element.

The Earth element helps us live into archetypes such as the Mother/Caretaker, the Gardener, and the Farmer. The Mama (male or female) nurtures the children, day after day. The Farmer gets up every single morning, takes the eggs from the chickens, milks the cows, and plows the fields. That's a lot of work, and a lot of devotion. Imagine a gardener who waters the plants and weeds the garden, cheerfully singing to their plant allies. Now, imagine the gardener that wakes up and says, "OMG, I can't believe I have to water these frickin' plants again!" That garden isn't going to last very long, and that gardener's bad attitude gives birth to another friend of the Earth element: *procrastination*. The Earth element gives us a healthy attitude adjustment when we experience resistance or overwhelm so that we can attend to our daily grind with patience, devotion, love, commitment, and humility.

Speaking of humility, these humble archetypes are not about showing off. There's not a lot of pomp and circumstance with the Earth element. I learned of this aspect as "tending to the dirt beneath my fingernails."[70] In other words:

---

70. Alchemical Mentorship Weekend Training Notes, Lorie Dechar, 2018.

the Earth is grounded and practical. It helps us take care of the stuff that's not so fun or inviting, but still has to get done. It's all about the work behind the scenes, the kind that doesn't get a lot of time in the spotlight. I mean, aside from the occasional highlight reel, the gardener doesn't post pictures of themselves watering the flowers every single day.

In the same way that the earth spins on its axis, when this aspect of Earth is out of balance, we may experience ideas that spin around and around in our heads. These ideas will never manifest if we don't birth them through action. Think of the person who says they are going to start a business, but ten years later, they are still talking about the business and haven't taken any steps to materialize their plan. The ideas are there, the excitement is there, the motivation might even be there. But for some reason, there's a disconnect between the ideas and the actual physical manifestation of them.

Every element in Chinese Medicine has a spiritual component, and the spirit of Earth is called *yi*. The glyph for *yi* is both poetic and powerful: It shows the character for "heart" underneath the character for "music," asking us, "Are we singing the song of our hearts?"[71] The *yi* of the Earth element helps us get out of a stuck place and is responsible for making sure our inspiration from heaven is empowered and animated with the energies of the earth. Step by step, things become real. The Earth element teaches us the way to manifest our dreams into reality: bit by bit, little by little, day by day.

The Earth element is there with us to keep us grounded and committed during the things that can't manifest overnight—like writing a book, losing twenty pounds, learning a new skill, or raising a decent human being. Some things require our dedication for weeks, months, years, or even lifetimes. We are here because of the sacrifices and choices of our mother's mothers' mothers. When we honor the mothers in the creative process, we honor the forces of devotion, nurturing, sacrifice, and commitment that allow us to exist.

Reflection Questions

How do you relate to the Mother archetype? Take a moment to reflect on the following questions in your journal:

71. Lorie Dechar, *Five Spirits: Alchemical Acupuncture for Psychological and Spiritual Healing* (Asheville, NC: Chiron Publications/Lantern Books, 2006), 218–219.

+ Who has played a mothering role for you?
+ What is your relationship with your mother? Your grandmothers?
+ What is your relationship with the earth?
+ How do you nurture yourself?
+ How do you feel about your responsibilities?
+ Who or what are you devoted to?
+ What in your life is calling for your committed, unwavering dedication?
+ What are the next, practical steps to realize your vision or goal?

Flower Essences to Honor the Mothers

The following flower essences help us to cultivate the qualities associated with archetypal Mother energy:

+ Mariposa Lily for nurturing and devotion
+ Quince for balancing strength and vulnerability
+ Tundra Rose for joyful commitment
+ Elm for attracting support

Mariposa Lily: A Mother's Embrace—Mariposa Lily is the quintessential essence for awakening and healing the mother archetype. When you hear the word "mother," what comes to mind? Media and pop culture give us so many options. Do you think of the mothers who seem to have it all together, like Jane Brady or Rainbow Johnson? Fiercely protective, ride-or-die mamas like the formidable Tasha St. Patrick? Do you picture Queen Bey and her pregnant belly with li'l Blue Ivy in tow? What about the Kris Jenner, Marge Simpson, and Angelina Jolie variations of mamahood?

Let's just pause for a moment to consider the magnitude of this most ancient archetype that has evolved over millennia. Embedded deeply in our psyche is an idea of what "mother" is and is not. Never has there been an archetype that has been so venerated, celebrated, and demonized. It is an archetype ladled with mythos, from the smiling sweet mother to the evil stepmother.

In her book *Archetypes: A Beginner's Guide to Your Inner-Net*, Carolyn Myss writes about the evolution of the Mom archetype in the Western world:

> The instant someone tells you that a woman is a *Perfect Mom*, you immediately picture a great cook with a charming, well-ordered home, who helps their kids with homework attends all their sporting events,

listens to their problems, hosts sleepovers with friends and bakes brownies. Even if the words *Perfect Mom* bring up painful associations with a not-so-perfect upbringing, you still have the projection of the ideal Mother figure firmly planted in your psyche.[72]

What's wonderful about Mariposa Lily flower essence is that it helps us reconcile the gap between the deified qualities of the Mother archetype— unconditional love, always giving, always nurturing and compassionate—and the reality of the mother we experience on earth. In real life, mothers are human. That means mothers make mistakes while healing from their own traumas and do the best they can without a manual or a learner's permit. Some of us have beautiful, harmonious relationships with our mothers or our children. Others have painful relationships that are distant, estranged, full of conflict, or nonexistent. Mariposa Lily flower essence helps us to reconcile the pain, guilt, shame, and wounding we may feel as we consider the role of the Mother archetype in life. It helps to bring compassion to the mother-child relationship. This flower essence facilitates awareness and the healing of core, unresolved wounds. Through this healing, we experience the Mother archetype as our innate capacity to nurture others as well as ourselves.

I love the show *This Is Us*, because it is one of the most honest portrayals of the mother-daughter relationship I have ever seen. Social media is full of "best friend" depictions of moms and daughters who wear matching outfits. Then there's the occasional "check on your mom friends with strong willed daughters—we are not okay" social media message that both evokes a laugh and strikes a painful chord. *This Is Us* explores both sides of this complicated dynamic. Through Kate and Rebecca, we see that motherhood is not always joyful—sometimes it is full of pain and contradictions, permeated with love that can be misinterpreted. I tearfully watch some episodes wondering what would happen if Mariposa Lily came to bless this fictional duo.

Mariposa Lily helps to ease the disillusion and the expectations that fray the bonds of mother and child. It opens communication and connection in all parent-child relationships. I often call on this remedy whenever a client needs to re-constellate their relationship with their children, especially during

---

72. Caroline Myss, *Archetypes: A Beginner's Guide to Your Inner-Net* (Carlsbad, CA: Hay House, 2014), 2.

times of transition: conception to pregnancy, pregnancy to newborn, newborn to toddler, toddler to school age, adolescent to teenager, teenager to young adult. These transitional stages often require the terms of the parent-child contract to be renegotiated, and Mariposa Lily eases the way. It's very useful postpartum, as new parents (both mothers and fathers) face feelings of overwhelm and feeling "not good enough" in their new role. Mariposa Lily is also helpful for parents who feel distant or unable to emotionally connect to their children.

No matter what stage we are at in our development or what our relationship with our mothers may be, Mariposa Lily offers sweetness and compassion into the relationship with those that gave us life, and with those we gave life. Even if we do not have access to our mothers in the physical world due to death, estrangement, or physical distance, Mariposa Lily helps to bring awareness and healing to this most primal relationship.

Mariposa Lily supports the positive activation of all variations of the Mother archetype, including the Caregiver, the Nurturer, the Teacher, the Rescuer, and the Healer. This flower essence is an ally for anyone who needs support offering loving, responsive, nurturing presence to help something or someone develop. Though aligned with the Sacred Feminine, this quality does not only manifest through women. Mariposa Lily is a beautiful, delicate flower that teaches us about the capacity of nurturing for the human soul.

A closely related species of this beautiful flower, Splendid Mariposa Lily, helps us honor the gift of life and also tap into the forces of nurturing we can receive from our primordial mothers. Splendid Mariposa Lily connects us to forces like Yemoja, a powerful deity of the Yoruba pantheon who is caretaker of all children. The ancient stories tell us that the earth's oceans, rivers, and streams manifested when Yemoja's waters broke. All life is nurtured in Yemoja's womb. We can also honor Gaia, the primordial personification of the earth in Greek mythology, and Asase Yaa, the great female spirit of the earth in the Akan tradition. These ancient and cosmic mothers are still here to guide, nurture, and comfort us.

Quince: Loving Strength and Vulnerability—Though most known for its edible fruit, quince is part of the rose family. Like all roses, it has an affinity for matters of the heart. However, unlike the delicate petals of the common rose, the pink petals of a quince blossom are thick and hearty. Quince reminds us that love requires strength. It helps us say, "I love you but *no*" and assert the boundaries and discipline necessary for nurturing and caring relationships.

On the A-train subway from Brooklyn to Manhattan, there used to be a poster with a low angle of a Black mama, hands on hips, with a fierce expression on her face. The caption read, "She doesn't love to be tough—she's tough because she loves." Unfortunately, this is a stereotypical image of Black motherhood—the mother who doesn't put up with any nonsense and has a tough hand. She is the brunt of jokes and condemnation. She accepts no backtalk and is swift to issue discipline, like Tachina Arnold's portrayal of Rochelle in the sitcom *Everybody Hates Chris* (actually one of my favorite mamas of all time!). I don't know any mamas who live out this caricature in real life. The real mamas I know wrestle with how to be both assertive and receptive, authoritative yet understanding.

Quince is one of my favorite essences for my mama clients who have to be both the primary nurturer and the primary disciplinarian. This role is not only overwhelming, it can also be confusing! Most folks will vacillate from being too strict about some matters and too lenient about others. Quince helps strike a balance between flexibility and resolve; tough love versus a gentle nudge in the right direction.

Quince flower essence affirms the strength needed to allow those we love to experience the consequences of their actions. It can also bring gentleness and sensitivity to the disciplinarian who is too harsh in their execution of justice. The parenting archetype incudes the Mama Bird, who goes off searching for worms, brings them back to the nest, and gently offers the food into the babies' li'l beaks. This is a role that requires sensitivity and care. But the mama bird also drop-kicks those babies out of the nest when it's time. It takes a certain amount of heart strength and resolve to love someone enough to let them fall in order to fly. Quince awakens insight into how to set the stage for fair, loving boundaries and consequences.

Quince reminds us that when we set a boundary, we don't have to do it with yelling, screaming, or angst. We can just say *no*. I remember my first conference with my daughter's second grade teacher. When I asked the teacher for a copy of an assignment, she sweetly said "no" in the gentlest voice. There was such a disconnect between her affect and her words that I thought I heard wrong! When I asked a second time, it was clear that her "no" was final. And that was that.

Quince helps us to integrate power with softness in all relationships. My girlfriend Khalilah, a bawse in every aspect of her short life, was a force to be reckoned with. She commanded attention in every space she entered and asserted an authority that was nonnegotiable. This served her well in her career, where she unapologetically confronted systemic racism in education. But what I will most remember Khalilah for is not for her work in the community. Nope! What I remember most is her heart.

Khalilah taught me the most important lesson of Quince flower essence: how to navigate being a woman who stands in her power and yet still is open to love. We talked often about how as Black women, we sometimes don't feel like we have the right, the privilege, or the tools to balance all that power in the outer world with all that vulnerability in our most intimate spaces. Spaces where we don't have control. Spaces where we don't have the answers. Spaces where we need help that we don't know how to ask for, let alone receive. I'm pretty convinced that Khalilah came into my life to teach me how to be, as she called it:

Soft n' pink

Warm 'n bubbly

Vulnerable 'n naive

It was Khalilah's couch that I laid on for seven straight days during the hardest part of my divorce. And it was Khalilah who I called on the verge of panic, before my first post-divorce date. She advised me to "be on time and have that lipstick poppin'!" Which still remains the most solid dating advice I've had to date.

Tundra Rose: Joyful Commitment—For my fortieth birthday, I completed a forty-day hot yoga challenge. By the end, I felt like a superwoman. My back was lengthened and tall. Instead of slumping my shoulders as per usual, I walked with my heart extended forward—vulnerable, exposed, and unafraid. I felt energy in parts of my body that were once numb and uninhabited. Even my ovaries were talking. I started the yoga challenge with a grandiose declaration: "I'm tired of feeling sluggish and relying on coffee. I am going to transform my health!" My Spirit Self said, "Hey, why don't you do a forty-day yoga challenge?" "Yes!" My Earth Self replied. And then together, we got all excited. I pictured myself strong and flexible after the challenge. I could see myself in cute colorful yoga outfits. I could hear my friends asking me how I did it. I could even see myself celebrating my success with a party. A big party for me! Yay me!

Our vision and excitement (thank you, Wood and Fire!) are enough to get us motivated, and even sometimes enough to get us started. But they don't sustain us through the process. Eventually our excitement fades and our vision gets blurry as we come to terms with the monotonous, mundane commitment that goes into nurturing a baby, a project, or a bright idea. Like a forty-day yoga challenge.

Tundra Rose helps us to value and lean into the tedious, unsexy, and often undesirable choices every day that make a vision become reality. For my yoga challenge, that included wrapping my head around:

- waking up at 5 am when the 6 am class was the only one that fit in my day
- drinking what felt like a bazillion gallons of water so I didn't pass out on the mat (it was actually only one gallon, but still)
- dragging a sleepy child still in pajamas to a yoga studio on a Saturday morning (pre-COVID)
- old leggings and tank tops with holes (instead of the sexy yoga clothes in my mind's eye)
- laundry … lots and lots of frickin' laundry

Tundra Rose supports us through the monotony of laborious, overwhelming, and uncelebrated tasks that happen behind the scene. For every kid we see thanking their mama at their high school graduation, we know there were approximately 6,570 days—some good and some awful—that went into that moment. For every book we read, thousands of hours went into writing, dreaming, visioning, typing, and correcting every typo and missing comma (Shout out to the Copy Qween, Logan Gamble, and my entire team at Llewellyn Worldwide!). Tundra Rose was a tremendous ally for my client, whose heart was heavy from the incessant responsibilities of cooking, cleaning, and hours on the phone with the insurance company after her partner suffered a traumatic injury.

In the Disney version of the fairy tale "Snow White," the seven dwarves kept their hearts light and playful by whistling while they worked. Similarly, Tundra Rose's beautiful yellow color brings joy to the heart as we take care of our responsibilities and handle our business. This feeling is the essence of devotion, and tundra rose supports joyous, committed service offered with love.

Elm: Systems of Support—Envision a beautiful, strong elm tree, mightily standing on its own. When we perceive Elm's individual strength, we are actually witnessing strength that is nurtured by community. In *The Hidden Life of Trees*, Peter Wohlleben describes the intricate, invisible systems of connection and communication between trees in a forest. Every tree has unique requirements for soil, light, water, and so on, yet the trees support each other by balancing out the distribution of their nutrients so that they can all thrive.

> The rate of photosynthesis is the same for all the trees. The trees, it seems, are equalizing differences between the strong and the weak. This equalization is taking place underground through the roots. There's obviously a lively exchange going on down there. Whoever has an abundance of sugar hands some over, whoever is running short gets help ... "A chain is only as strong as its weakest link." Because trees know this intuitively, they do not hesitate to help each other out.[73]

Wohllenben goes on to share the many ways that trees communicate with one another through a science that is beyond our ordinary perception. For example, when a giraffe starts chomping on leaves of an acacia tree, the tree sends a message through its roots to its neighbors. They respond by releasing a toxic chemical into their leaves, which the giraffe senses and moves on about its business to continue grazing a hundred meters away. A tree that loses its ability to communicate with its comrades due to sickness or trauma is the first to get infested with insects. From the fungi to the roots, the natural world has truly magical ways to communicate with, depend on, and support one another. Elm teaches us what these trees have known from the beginning: we are better together.

---

73. Peter Wohlleben, *The Hidden Life of Trees: What They Feel, How They Communicate: Discoveries from a Secret World* (New York: HarperCollins, 2020), 25–27.

Elm flower essence opens our receptivity to support so that we may also be nurtured by community. It resonates closely with the Hero archetype, which is activated in a person who feels a strong compulsion to save the day. They will be the first to volunteer for a task that needs to be done, and will often effectively and single-handedly manage the many tasks that keep a household, company, or project operating smoothly. The person who benefits from Elm will consciously or unconsciously believe that they don't need or deserve help. This flower essence allows us to release the pressure of those internal and external expectations. It helps us to be realistic and responsive to the demands in front of us and clear about what we actually have the capacity to take on.

Elm helps us reorganize what's on our plate, to take stock and to say, "Okay, *this* I don't actually have to do; I can release control and allow someone else to step in, in this instance." Or it helps us say, "Oh, you know there *is* a person I can ask for help. I don't have to do this by myself." I consider Elm flower essence an ally that supports what Caroline Myss identifies as the call of the Caretaker archetype:

+ consciously decide when and how to care for someone
+ care for others out of compassion, never guilt or obligation
+ take care of yourself so that you have the physical, emotional, and spiritual stamina to care for others
+ fully own your destiny to be there for others[74]

A person who needs Elm flower essence will begin to reflect on the compulsive ways in which they take on new tasks and projects, as well as what can be taken off their plate. Elm also offers permission to receive help and fosters awareness of the limiting beliefs that become blocks to receiving support. Maybe we believe it would take too much energy or time to teach someone how to help, or perhaps there is a fear that we will be let down by others if we depend on them. Or, our ego—accustomed to being the Healer or Rescuer—leads us to believe that we are the only or best person for the job. Elm helps to dismantle the myth that we have to go at it alone, and allows us to receive that support from wherever it might be coming from. Often, the support we need is already around us—all we have to do is ask.

---

74. Myss, *Archetypes*, 101.

Embodied Practice: Malasana (Deep Squat Pose)

Affirmation: I birth it, I nurture it, I allow it.

Begin by standing with your feet slightly wider than hip-width apart, toes angled outward. Slowly bend your knees, drawing your hips toward the floor. Feel free to place pillows, blankets, or blocks under your tailbone so that you can hold the position comfortably. Bring your hands together in prayer position, gently resting elbows on your knees or using them to widen your squat. If you can do so without creating strain, lower your heels toward the ground. Lengthen your spine as you lift the crown of your head toward the sky while sinking your hips toward the earth.

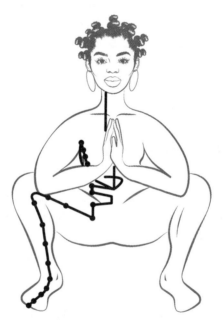

Pictured with the Spleen Meridian

As you assume the position of the great cosmic mothers of creation, call to mind what you want to manifest. Envision yourself birthing it into the universe.

Repeat the affirmation: *I birth it, I nurture it, I allow it.*

Take a moment to honor the mothers, the creative forces of the manifested world.

Soul Lesson 2: Find Your Center

When you say "yes" to others,
make sure you are not saying "no" to yourself.
—Paulo Coelho

We often think of fire and water as opposites. Yet, the Wood element and the Earth element form an equally dynamic polarity. The Wood element asserts, "Do *you*, Boo!" while Earth element asks, "What about us?" Wood pushes us to stand solidly in our vision and personal perspective, while Earth teaches us how to compromise and consider the perspectives of others. Wood celebrates individualism and self-actualization, while Earth celebrates family and community. The two are as polarized as capitalism and communism.

The Earth-Wood polarity shows up in so many ways. As a mom, I struggle to balance my personal needs with the needs of my family. Others wrestle with choices such as going into the family business versus following their own dreams. And in our daily interactions, we may be challenged with how to meet our own needs while also considering the group's needs. If I don't honor my individuality, I sacrifice my integrity. But if I don't honor my community, I lose my sense of connection. What do we do with the doubt, guilt, fear, or worry that greets us when we decide to put ourselves first? What do we do with the resentment that simmers when we agree to put ourselves last? These two aspects of our psyche are in constant negotiation, trying to balance one another. The Earth element supports us as we navigate a successful balance between you, me, and we.

One of the most common African proverbs is *Ubuntu*, which is often translated as "I am because we are, and we are because I am." It is a word from the Nguni peoples of southern Africa. In the Xhosa language, the proverb is expressed as *Ubuntu ungamntu ngabanya abantu*, and in Zulu, *Umuntu ngumuntu ngabanye*. It means "my humanity is caught up and inextricably bound up in the humanity of others," or "a person is a person through other people."[75]

---

75. Chioma Ohajunwa and Gubela Mji, "The African Indigenous Lens of Understanding Spirituality: Reflection on Key Emerging Concepts from a Reviewed Literature," *Journal of Religion and Health* 57, no. 6 (2018): 2523–2537.

In the traditional African worldview, there is no individual success if the collective suffers. And the health of the community is dependent upon the success of each of its individuals. We are interconnected. This means that yes, I am an individual. My individuality—my unique purpose and gifts—contribute to the wholeness of my family and community. But I would not have a unique purpose or individual gifts were it not for the support of my community. The individual and the community are two sides of a single coin. You can't have one without the other.

A *synecdoche* is a part of speech in which the part represents the whole and vice versa: we mention the "ABCs" to refer to the whole alphabet; we count "heads" when tallying a number of people; and when we talk about our "wheels," we mean the whole car. Similarly, when you see me as an individual, I represent a collective. When you see a collective, it should also represent me. Rather than true opposites, Wood and Earth complement one another.

Classical acupuncture texts teach us that sympathy and overthinking are associated with the Earth element. In my experience, a better description would be sympathetic resonance. We see sympathetic resonance in action when an opera singer shatters a wineglass, which happens because the pitch and the frequency of the singer's voice is resonant with the frequency of the glass. Similarly, when two guitars are perfectly tuned, a C string plucked on one guitar will cause the C string on the other to vibrate. This type of sympathetic resonance also happens in heart-to-heart connections. When something tugs on one person's heartstring, another person's heartstring vibrates in resonance. For example, if we are next to someone weeping, it strikes a chord within our hearts and we feel empathy.

The Earth element allows us to feel with, vibe with, and tune in to the emotions of those we care for as part of an interconnected field of energy. With compassion and sympathy, we feel each other's feels. When I see pain in the world, that pain strikes a chord within me. And when I see joy in the world, that joy strikes a chord within me. Some of us have too much sensitivity to other people's chords and some of us don't have enough.

In *The Art of Empathy, a Complete Guide to Life's Most Essential Skill*, emotional expert Karla McLaren describes hyperempathy and its six essential aspects, all of which can be supported by nourishing the Earth element:

1. Emotional Contagion: Tthe capacity to sense, acknowledge, and feel emotions in an environment. In hyperempaths, emotional contagion leads a person to sometimes confuse another person's feeling with their own.
2. Empathic Accuracy: the ability to accurately identify and understand emotional states, thoughts and intentions in yourself and others.
3. Emotional Regulation: self-awareness and the ability to work with your own emotional states, as well as function skillfully in the presence of strong emotions.
4. Perspective Taking: the ability to put yourself in the place of others, to understand what they want or need.
5. Concern for others: the ability to engage with others in a way that shows care and compassion.
6. Perceptive Engagement: The ability to act or respond to the needs of others.[76]

The flower essences and soul medicine practices introduced in this section will help you recognize when emotional contagion is happening, as well as cultivate the skills necessary to successfully relate to others from your own center. We are separate physical beings, yet we are energetically connected. The Earth element supports us as we feel into one another and respond with love, care, and clear energetic boundaries. This is how we honor the connection of shared human experience.

Reflection Questions

Are you centered and grounded in yourself? Take a moment to reflect on the following questions in your journal:

+ How do you balance caring for yourself and caring for others?
+ How easy is it for you to feel the feels of someone else? Is this healthy or imbalanced?
+ How do you create loving boundaries?
+ How do you show care and concern for those around you? Do you have a sensitive presence?

---

76. Karla McLaren, *The Art of Empathy: A Complete Guide to Life's Most Essential Skill* (Louisville, CO: Sounds True, 2013), 26–27.

+ What gifts to you bring to your family or community? What gifts
  does your family or community bring to you?

Flower Essences to Find Your Center

The flower essences in this section are my favorites to support our capacity for healthy empathy, in a way that honors both the individual and the collective:

+ Pink Yarrow to build an emotional force field
+ Yellow Star Tulip to cultivate compassionate connection
+ Indian Pink to bring calm in the midst of chaos
+ Red Chestnut to settle a worried heart

Pink Yarrow: Build an Emotional Force Field—Yarrow is a sturdy plant known for its protective nature. It looks like a cluster of tiny umbrellas that shield us from the turbulent elements. The plant's scientific name is *Achillea millefolium*, and you may notice a reference to the name of the Trojan War hero in Greek mythology. Legends tell us that Achilles was dipped into a bath of yarrow for protection in battle and also used the plant to treat his soldier's wounds. Yarrow helps us to form an energetic force field around us so that we can be centered, grounded, and clear.

The three most common varieties of yarrows are pink, white, and golden. Pink Yarrow creates an emotional boundary around the heart, allowing us to clearly distinguish our feelings from the feelings of others. It helps us cultivate emotional accuracy and emotional regulation, especially when there are too many emotions clouding the energetic boundaries between self and other. This is my go-to flower essence for hyperempaths, who feel off-centered by the strong emotions of others and often mistake them as their own. As children, they develop extraordinary perception of the emotional climate of those around them, possibly to brace themselves for bullying, abuse, or other negative behaviors that overwhelm their inherent sensitivity. Hyperempaths may also have challenges asserting boundaries, as they intuitively recoil from an anticipated or perceived reaction.

What's beautiful about this flower essence is that rather than muting or numbing our sensitivity, it supports us in maximizing the gift of etheric sensitivity. When I suspect that a patient's anxiety may be calmed with Pink Yarrow flower essence, I often ask about their relationship with pets or plants.

Just as these individuals can easily experience the emotions of fellow humans, they can feel calmed and supported by plant, mineral, and animal allies in the natural world. Their sensitivity to subtle energetic influences opens them to effortlessly experience the energetic qualities of gemstones, essential oils, and natural landscapes.

As a habitual hyperempath, one of my favorite exercises when I need Pink Yarrow's support is a practice I call the *Hubba Bubba Bubble* (no judgment!). This quick inner visualization helps me get immediate insight into any emotional contagion in the field. I begin by taking a deep breath to steady myself. I close my eyes and envision a bright-pink-yarrow-colored bubble surrounding me. Like bubblegum (hence the name), the walls of the bubble are thick enough to keep me nurtured and safe yet translucent enough for me to see everything and everyone around me.

Next, I call to mind the person with whom I am relating. If that person appears in my mind's eye *inside* the bubble with me, I know there is an energetic boundary that needs reinforcement. It alerts me that I am confusing their desires, expectations, needs, or pain with my own. In my imaginal sight, I gently place this person on the outside of my bubble's walls, where I can still see and interact with them lovingly. Once this image is clear (sometimes it takes a while to move someone up and out of my bubble!), I can better distinguish their needs from my own. Often, this meditation will surface insight into how to effectively communicate or respond to the situation in question.

Pink Yarrow helps us build a soft, translucent energetic bubble around the heart to shield us from emotional enmeshment or a contagion. Once this protection is in place, we can sit next to the experience of someone else without taking it on for ourselves. We can clearly distinguish our own feelings, while remaining present to the feelings of others. In addition, Pink Yarrow supports our ability to ask about what we are sensing from others to make sure that our perceptions of their feelings are even accurate to begin with. From this place of clarity and discernment, we can relate to others from our own emotional and energetic center.

Yellow Star Tulip: Compassionate Connection—If Pink Yarrow is the flower essence we turn to for hyperempathy and emotional contagion, Yellow Star Tulip supports the opposite end of the empathy spectrum—this essence reminds us that there is a difference between centering the self and being self-centered. It refines our ability to see ourselves in another person's shoes, and to respond with concern. The person who needs Yellow Star Tulip is often so centered in their own solar plexus energy that they lack sensitivity to their environment. This includes the feelings and emotions of others, as well as nonverbal social cues. They may come across as cold or harsh, offering little to no compassion. In other cases, the person needing Yellow Star Tulip will try to empathize with another person's experience but somehow end up talking about themselves. Their expression of "I know exactly how you feel…" becomes a conversational pivot to their own experience rather than an expression of compassion. Sounds like an unlikeable person, right? Wrong! Sometimes the Yellow Star Tulip soul is quite lovable.

Abed Nadir, a character played by Danny Pudi on the television sitcom *Community*, is extraordinarily perceptive of and attuned to the concrete, practical world. Yet, he demonstrates a profound inability to read social cues and make emotional connections. He tends to see the world only through his eyes, which is typical of someone who would benefit from Yellow Star Tulip. Jeff Winger, the show's self-involved narcissist, played by Joel McHale, could also use a little Yellow Star Tulip. His character illustrates how the boisterous and charismatic personality of a person needing this flower essence can often naturally make them shine as the leader or life of the party. Throughout the six seasons (and a movie!) of *Community*, both Abed and Jeff became increasingly sensitive, thoughtful, and responsive to their colleagues' emotional needs. Yellow Star Tulip would be so proud!

Like many bright yellow flowers that illuminate our shadowy parts, Yellow Star Tulip's negative tendencies are easier to see in others than in ourselves. If we are in conflicts where we are frequently accused of not understanding other points of view, Yellow Star Tulip may be in order. If you happen to notice that people fall silent when you start talking or that fewer friends confide in you, you might want to introduce Yellow Star Tulip and observe how your relationships shift. We can also consider Yellow Star Tulip if we feel unusually numb to others' pain in suffering. Rolling your eyes or thinking "here we go again" when that friend calls you with her thousandth crisis may be a sign that your emotional sensitivity is burned out.

Yellow Star Tulip is a primary essence I turn to for therapists and healers who are experiencing emotional fatigue and burn-out that leads to apathy in the treatment room. I also recommend this essence to parents who, perhaps due to overwhelm and exhaustion, need support attuning to the needs of their children. Yellow Star Tulip helps us reengage with emotional presence without losing our own center. In environments that require collaboration and teamwork, Yellow Star Tulip can increase our sensitivity to the spoken and unspoken needs of the group. As we extend our awareness beyond our personal needs and perspectives, we are better positioned to negotiate winwin resolutions.

In most cases, we don't need Yellow Star Tulip because we are inherently selfish. Instead, this flower essence can support us when we are, as McLaren describes, hyperempaths who are simply burnt out from not being able to manage heightened emotional sensitivity in the past.[77] In this case, Yellow Star Tulip gently reawakens our soul sensitivity. As this sensitivity awakens, we feel more attuned to the needs of others, as well as more connected as part of the human family.

Indian Pink: Calm though Chaos—Recall a time when you were surrounded by a million things on your to-do list, all calling for your urgent attention. There are past-due deadlines and bills. There are projects left demanding completion. The kitchen is a mess with dirty dishes and takeout containers because you haven't had the time to cook. You finally clear out some space to get some work done … and then the phone rings. A family member is in crisis, and you need to drop everything to lend your support. This is a classic Indian Pink scenario.

Indian Pink flower essence helps us find the center of the whirlwind storm that is the chaos of our lives. From the eye of this storm, we can see clearly all the things whirling around us and prioritize and organize a plan to bring some calm to the chaos. It supports the empathic skill of emotional regulation, through which we are able function skillfully in our best interests while feeling strong emotions. When Indian Pink is an ally, those strong emotions can include excitement, sympathy, grief, overwhelm, worry, or fear—anything that rocks the boat or rocks our world.

On a mundane level, Indian Pink helps us get our life together. Instead of seeing a confusing pile of tasks, Indian Pink will help us with a clear sense of

---

77. McLaren, *The Art of Empathy*, 36–38.

how to get organized. We gain insight into exactly how to order our steps: "I'm going to do this first. I'm going to do this second. I'm going to do this third. I'm not going to do this at all. This isn't important. This is a distraction." Indian Pink helps us to see patterns and priorities. This brings us out of our chaos-induced paralysis and into taking clear and deliberate action.

On a spiritual level, Indian Pink is an ally when it seems like everything is falling apart at the same time. There are those transformational moments when all the supports we were leaning on suddenly start crumbling. One catastrophe leads to another, and before we know it, everything is out of control. Our life feels like absolute chaos and we can't seem to get our footing. Indian Pink helps us come back to a steady center. It also has a very calming and settling effect on the spirit. Where we might have previously felt overwhelmed, we feel centered and serene, just like the eye of the tornado.

Red Chestnut: A Settled Heart—Like White Chestnut (see the Metal chapter), Red Chestnut settles the mind and quiets the heart. This is the flower essence that we call on when we are consumed with worry about someone else's well-being, safety, or happiness. Worry drives us to do the absolute most, which—though coming from good intentions—is very annoying for those on the receiving end. The Red Chestnut state can manifest as overprotection, manipulation, or helicoptering.

Picture a new mother fretting over her baby: "Does he have enough clothes? Is he warm enough? Is he cool enough? Is he lying on his back? Is he lying on his stomach?" When I was a new mom, I would wake up in the middle of the night to make sure my child was breathing, covering her nose until she stirred. The hypervigilant feeling to protect the vulnerability of an infant is natural. But sometimes, this natural Earth element ability gets turned on its head and goes into overdrive. Think of the mother who still treats their thirty-year-old child as if they're a toddler, trying to micromanage their life, or becoming consumed with thoughts about their safety. This dynamic can emerge in any relationship where we feel responsible for the well-being of someone we love.

Red Chestnut comes into the picture when we are consciously or subconsciously playing God as we try to manipulate experiences for the person we care about. This includes trying to keep them from experiencing pain, discomfort, or inconvenience. In this state, we go to extraordinary measures so that a loved one can feel safe and can have what they need. As a result, we feel anxiety, sometimes on their behalf.

Here's an example: My mom was in a car accident last August and needed several surgeries during her recovery. Separated by COVID and a couple hundred miles, I was so worried! I called her every five minutes, pestering her with questions: "Did you go to the doctor? What did they say? Did you do this? Did you do that?" Finally, my mom exclaimed, "Can you please stop worrying about me!? I'm a grown-ass woman. I've got this!" When Red Chestnut is called for, our worry will make us overstep another's boundaries, agency, and personal power. If you are doing the most for someone and they respond with irritation instead of gratitude, check yourself before you wreck yourself! Their frustration (Wood element) may be a sign that your Earth element is out of balance. Red Chestnut gently coaches us from the sidelines and reminds us: "You know … this is actually not your jurisdiction. Allow some space for this person to walk their own path. Their own spiritual power and spiritual supports are part of the equation." Worry and anxiety can then give way to a deep and profound trust in their freedom and agency.

Family Constellations therapy—a system developed by Bert Hellinger after studying the philosophies of the Zulu nation—illustrates this principle. In Family Constellation therapy, one technique is to guide clients through an embodied visualization of their loved one surrounded by a web of visible support from family, community, and invisible allies in the spiritual world. Similarly, Red Chestnut awakens the understanding that our loved ones come with a support system that extends beyond our capacity to be everyone and do everything for them. This realization brings a sense of relief, and a more balanced approach to offering care and concern.

I use this flower often with patients who are caretakers, a role that is often steeped with worry and anxiety. There can also be a lot of fear that comes with the territory. Red Chestnut helps to quiet the heart so that there can be a calm distance between our concern and our anxiety. With Red Chestnut, worry is replaced with trust and faith that the person is supported and has the physical and/or spiritual resources they need. It is a great remedy for parents, especially in stages where children are beginning to assert their independence and autonomy. It is useful for those in romantic relationships who are worried about their lovers. It can help anyone who obsessively worries about how someone they love is moving through the world and what they might experience along the way.

Red Chestnut flower essence doesn't absolve us of our responsibilities as caretakers, but it does help dissipate the anxiety and fear that come with the role. It supports healthy perspective taking, a skill that requires emotional empathy. As we gain a healthy perspective, our empathy and actions can come from compassion and wisdom instead of from fear. Through this discernment, we attune to how we can appropriately support the needs of those we love.

Embodied Practice: Ardha Matsyendrasana (Half Lord of the Fishes Pose)

Affirmation: I turn to others from my own center.

Begin by sitting with both legs extended in front of you. Tenderly bend your left knee, offering self-care and love as you hug it toward your chest. Gently lift your left foot, crossing it over your right leg and placing it on the floor next to your right knee. Use your left hand for balance on the floor next to your hip as you twist at the waist toward your left. Press your right elbow against the inside of your knee to deepen the twist.

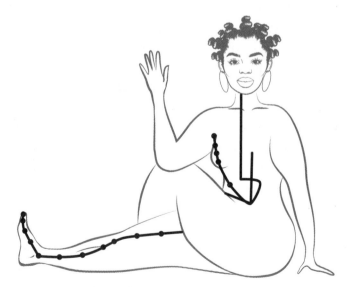

Pictured with the Spleen Meridian

Envision yourself interacting lovingly with others while feeling grounded and supported. Close your eyes and repeat the affirmation: *I turn to others from my own center.*

Reverse your legs and repeat the twist on the opposite side.

Soul Lesson 3: Your Body Is a Temple

We are not human beings having a spiritual experience;
we are spiritual beings having a human experience.
—Pierre Teilhard de Chardin

Western medicine as we know it today is based on the Western biomedicine model, which asserts that only what can be measured matters. Because *matter matters*, if we can find an observable cause of illness or disease (such as a virus, infection, or organic dysfunction), we can find a cure by eradicating that source. Advanced medical technologies have developed to increase our capacity to see and objectively measure causative agents in the human body. The scientific goal is to discover, name, and ultimately control more and more of the observable universe.

Biomedicine uses diagnostic methods that extend our five senses to discover the cause of pain or disease, whether by sight (including MRIs, X-rays, blood work, or other imaging studies), sound (including sonograms, stethoscopes, and so on), touch (muscle tension or lesions in the skin), and so on. We look for materialized phenomenon that can be identified as the cause of illness.

There is a tremendous amount of expertise in conventional medicine to serve the physical body. The technology is amazing, and I'm all for knowing everything there is for us to know about healing. But what about the patients whose illness can't be diagnosed? What does a medicine for the physical body know of heartache, grief, or the healing power of laughter? Biomedicine asserts that the world we can perceive through our five senses is more real or valid than what we perceive through intuition, feeling, and spirit. In addition, Western biomedicine has been historically hostile to Black and Brown bodies, from the treatment of Sarah Baartman to the Tuskegee experiments. The book *Medical Apartheid: The Dark History of Medical Experimentation on Black Americans from Colonial Times to Present* documents the many ways in which Black and Brown bodies have been traumatized by so-called scientific advancement.[78]

The health industry is based on a standard of white male physiology, and though that's changing, it's not changing nearly fast enough. Even something as ordinary and everyday as the BMI (Body Mass Index) has dangerous implications. Do you know how many Black women are told they are obese, when they are in fact quite healthy thick chicks? Even worse, how many Black and Brown women are sent back out into the world with our depression and weight gain, dismissed because our thyroid levels fall within the ranges considered normal…for a 150-pound white man? Or consider Serena Williams's heart-wrenching childbirth story, which illustrates the need for women of color to be our own best health advocates and to know our bodies and souls intimately. As a result, many of us look at our doctors' recommendations with a serious and well-deserved Michelle Obama side-eye (Google "Michelle Obama at Trump inauguration" and you'll see exactly the kind of fierce side-eye I'm talking about).

I was diagnosed with premature menopause in my early twenties. It meant that I could not have children naturally—never, ever, ever Amen. My blood work results showed all the things that you absolutely don't want to see when you are trying to get pregnant: this hormone level is way too high, that hormone level is way too low. I consulted doctor after doctor, looking for someone to affirm that it was possible for me to defy the 1 percent odds of natural conception. I finally found a holistic OB-GYN, and shared with her the impossibly high FSH levels in my most recent blood work. She smiled and said, "Yes, but your body's different every day." She reminded me that the blood work was just a snapshot of where my body was at that moment the blood was taken.

That conversation completely shifted my perspective and initiated my journey to learning, studying, embracing, and celebrating a simple truth: *everything changes*. When the Greek philosopher Heraclitus declared that the only thing constant is change, he wasn't kidding. He was also restating a principle

---

78. Harriet A. Washington, *Medical Apartheid: The Dark History of Medical Experimentation on Black Americans from Colonial Times to the Present* (New York: Anchor Books, 2008).

that is central to the Indigenous healing philosophies that are the backbone of complementary and alternative medicine. Indigenous people "saw the physical world as a reflection of a complex, subtler, and more lasting yet invisible entity called energy."[79] This principle, dynamism, means that everything is energy—and when I say everything, I mean *everything*. Even the densest rock is slowly moving energy. Dynamism explains that there is a part of our body outside of the range of what our five senses can detect, known as the subtle body. The subtle body is a continuum from the densest aspect of our bodies—our bones, flesh, and blood—all the way to the most ephemeral aspect of ourselves, which is our spirit. Everything is a frequency. Everything is a vibration, some of which we can perceive, most of which we can't. When we welcome the spirit of dynamism, every- and anything can change, no matter how rigid, permanent, or impossible it may seem.

Mind and body are not separate: they are a continuum such that our illness could be physical, mental, emotional, or circumstantial. If your relationship isn't working, your finances aren't right, or your home has a leak in the ceiling—all these events are a reflection of illness to the Indigenous way of thinking. Health is not just about what's happening with our bodies: we can have toxic thoughts; that's an illness. If we don't know our greatness, that's also an illness. The spirit touches all aspects of our being, and nature is an ally in that work.

The subtle body includes the physical body, allowing us to embrace all the miraculous technological advances of biomedicine. And understanding the subtle body also allows us to facilitate our healing and well-being on mental, emotional, and spiritual levels. Dynamism reminds us that our bodies can change, our circumstances can change, and our relationships can change. It's all energy, and it can *all* change. How? You guessed it! With the patience, dedication, devotion, and practical commitment of the Earth element. And how do we understand the process of change? Right again! Through observing the rhythms and cycles of nature.

---

79. Malidoma Patrice Somé, *The Healing Wisdom of Africa: Finding Life Purpose through Nature, Ritual, and Community* (London: Thorsons, 1999), 23.

Though distinct in practice, the Dagara, Lucumi, and Ifa traditions of the Africa Diaspora, Native American shamanism, East Asian medicine, Celtic rituals, and the ayurvedic system of India are just a few examples of nature-based healing systems that still thrive today. Each is a system to witness a reflection of the Divine expressed through nature. Our bodies are an extension of nature, and they are a reflection of the Divine.

Dr. Na'im Akbar, a pioneer in African psychology, has written extensively about the African understanding of the relationship between the psyche and nature. He explains that our ancestors revered nature because the cycles of growth, maturation and transformation are symbolic metaphors for our spiritual development.[80] The visible world is always a reflection of the invisible, and nature reflects the divine laws that govern the universe. On Earth, as it is in Heaven.

In 2016, I was invited to create a wellness program for youth in New York City's public schools. The program introduced high school students to the five elements as a template for personal development. This work has reassured me that though ancient, the elements are alive and well! In fact, many of the songs in the playlists in this book are recommendations from my students. We would end each class with call and response of mantras to honor the organic transformation of nature. I adapted these movements and mantras from my teacher, mentor, and friend Lorie Dechar:

> I Am (Water)
>
> I Become (Wood)
>
> I Love (Fire)
>
> I Nurture (Earth)
>
> I Matter (Metal)[81]

The Earth element reminds us to cultivate our bodies like a garden. Flowers respond to the sun, water, air, and love the same way that our bodies are recharged with sun, water, air, and love. We are nature. Cultivating a relation-

---

80. Na'im Akbar, *Know Thyself* (Tallahassee, FL: Mind Productions & Associates, 1999), 46–48.

81. Lorie Dechar Alchemical Healing Mentorship, 2012–2018, Used with permission.

ship with nature is cultivating a relationship with our innermost selves. The Earth element invites us to honor our physical bodies as holy temples for our spirit and soul.

Reflection Questions

Take a moment to check in with your body before reflecting on the following questions in your journal:

+ What foods do you find healing? Which create discomfort or imbalance?
+ What is exercise routine makes you feel strong and vibrant?
+ Which parts of your body feel ignored, numb, or uninhabited?
+ How do you connect to nature?
+ How do you tend to the needs of your body?

Flower Essences to Honor Your Body

The following flower essences support healing our physical bodies, and remind us that our bodies are a temple for the spirit:

+ Self-Heal to awaken your healing intelligence
+ Nicotiana to soften emotional and physical armoring
+ Manzanita to ground into your body

Self-Heal: Awaken Your Healing Intelligence—Imagine you get a nasty cut on your finger. You clean it off and then put on a bandage to keep anything from getting in there. It stings for a while before closing and forming a scab. When you look at your finger a few weeks later, you can barely see traces of that cut. Did your bandage heal your finger? Of course not! Your body has a blueprint of what your healthy finger looks like, and each skin cell on your finger is encoded with that blueprint. The bandage just created a protective barrier so that your body could safely do what it already knows how to do—and that's get to the business of healing.

In a similar way, Self-Heal flower essence helps us to create the optimal conditions for our body to heal on the physical, emotional, mental, and spiritual planes. Our bodies already know how to heal, and Self-Heal flower essence awakens that knowing in every cell. Our bodies are encoded with an innate healing intelligence, and we are invited to consciously create the conditions that encourage, support, and protect that healing. Healing is an inside job. But how can we tap into the intelligence of a body that already knows what it needs to be happy, healthy, and whole? Self-Heal flower essence leads the charge.

Self-Heal flower essence teaches us and inspires us to do what we need to do for ourselves to heal. You know daggone well that dairy gives you the bubble guts, but you eat that bowl of mac 'n cheese anyway. Or coffee gives you the jitters, but you still brew a cup every morning. You're no good with only five hours of sleep, yet it's 2 am and you're binge-watching a show you've seen a thousand times. You want to start your mornings with meditation, yet there you are, scrolling through your social media feeds as soon as you wake up. Self-Heal swoops in to shift your relationship with your health habits, so that you not only have the awareness, but also the motivation to change. Self-Heal can also release emotions or memories your body is holding to allow gentle exploration of the stressors underlying your symptoms, including insight into the people, habits, or situations that negatively impact your well-being.

A healer or doctor doesn't heal you, but they do help to create the conditions for you to heal yourself. This does not mean that when we work with Self-Heal flower essence, we can stop working with our health professionals and go it alone (please don't do that!). Through synchronicity, this essence can often lead us to the right practitioner to support our healing journey. Their advice may come in the form of medication, therapy, dietary suggestions, lifestyle changes, or energy practices. Self-Heal helps us to feel aligned with— rather than afraid of or resistant to—proper care and treatment.

Self-Heal also helps us to get insight into what exactly is going on in these crazy bodies of ours. I call Self-Heal the "Mystery Medicine." Often when my clients have this flower essence in their regimen, they will get a diagnosis that *finally* makes sense. They may have had confusing symptoms for months or even years; they've seen specialists and done their online research; they've tried every supplement or medication under the sun, yet their symptoms persist. With the help of Self-Heal, suddenly an either obscure or obvious solution emerges that then opens their pathway for healing.

Solving medical mysteries is a big part of Self-Heal's magic. As we design our personal wellness regimen, it can serve the role of problem-solver. Maybe you want to meditate, but you don't know how. You want to take a yoga class, but don't know what studio to go to. You're confused about which dietary advice to follow (there's so much out there!), or can't organize your evening so that you can be in bed by eleven p.m. Self-Heal comes in and helps you get your entire life together. Suddenly, you have insight into the exact time going to the gym can fit into your busy life, or the friends to invite on your morning walk. It cuts through the excuses and the limiting beliefs we create that keep us from adopting a healthier lifestyle.

Self-Heal is an ally for anyone who wants to be healthier but doesn't know what steps to take. It is equally beneficial to the person who wants to spruce up their health regimen as it is to the person navigating a debilitating disease. In circumstances when physical change is not possible, Self-Heal reminds us that we can be healthy and whole in spite of our physical limitations. Self-Heal empowers us with insight into our personal agency and awakens our healing intelligence and resilience.

Nicotiana: Soften the Armor—In 2009, I traveled to Nevada City, California to study flower essence therapy with Patricia Kaminski and Richard Katz, the founders of the Flower Essence Society. Patricia and Richard are extraordinary humans. The love, care, and devotion they put into cultivating the farming their seventeen-acre botanical garden flowers as well as the numerous philanthropic projects they initiate around the globe demonstrate the archetypal signatures of the Earth element. When I was at Terra Flora, my entire body opened to receive the wisdom of nature.[82] The time I spent conversing and hanging out with those flowers was life-changing. Then it was time to head back to New York. As the plane hovered over the clouds and began to descend into LaGuardia Airport, I could already feel the whimsical openness I had experienced in northern Cali harden into the armor that I needed to navigate the Brooklyn streets. I braced myself for the sirens, the

---

82. "Terra Flora" is the name of the biodynamic garden cultivated by the Flower Essence Society.

concrete, the noise, the pollution, the trash, and the crowds with a deep sadness in my heart. Environmental activist Carl Anthony describes my experience as the sense of loss suffered by many people living in the city who are traumatized by the fact that they don't have a functional relationship to nature.[83] I wept at the isolation and disconnection, experiencing my internal separation from paradise.

Nicotiana is the flower essence that addresses numbing and armoring to protect emotional sensitivity. It is a flowering tobacco plant native to North America, and it is the flower essence I call on when parts of the body seem to feel uninhabited or numb, including and especially the heart. Our body kindly locks and stores away emotions we are not ready to face, but over time this hardening results in a tough, impenetrable persona that is hardened to the essence of life.

The archetypal image of someone needing Nicotiana is the person leaning against a wall, smoking a cigarette with dark shades and an air that says, "I'm unfuck-with-able." Nicotiana helps dissolve the callous and tough exterior-defense mechanism that protects our vulnerability. The flower essence supports our ability to experience our emotions with authenticity and express ourselves with integrity. We become more in touch with our feelings instead of relying on a tough, hardened exterior to keep others away.

Whether we assume a tough exterior or harden our souls on the inside, Nicotiana is the flower essence that I turn to when we use any substance to help us avoid or quiet the intensity of uncomfortable feelings. Emotional eating is a real thing, and Nicotiana is an ally when we turn to alcohol, sugar, or rich comfort foods as anesthesia for our stress. The comfort we feel is temporary and serves to further devitalize our bodies in the long run. The body is sneaky—it knows that the less alive we feel, *the less we have to feel.* The same numbing mechanism is at work with smoking, particularly tobacco. Rather than chastise my clients with the negative health consequences of their cigarette habits (which they already know), I consider smoking their way of self-medicating to help calm the intensity of their feelings. I offer Nicotiana to

---

83. Andy Fisher, *Radical Ecopsychology: Psychology in the Service of Life* (New York: State University of New York Press, 2013), 20.

gently support their ability to face those stressors and triggers without relying on cigarettes as a numbing agent. Rather than focusing on the smoking, they are able to attune to what their soul is avoiding. Once they begin to address the underlying stress, the smoking habit becomes less enticing.

I've lived in an urban environment for more than twenty years, which I could not do without the help of this soulful flower essence. The hardness of NYC's concrete industrial buildings gives off the same "unfuckwithable" toughness and standoffish vibes. Green Nicotiana is one variety of nicotiana that specifically supports us as we develop a relationship to nature in a technological, urban environment. It also appropriately softens the numbness and tough exterior we put on to navigate city living. It was a benevolent friend to me as I reacclimated to New York after a week of spiritual opening, and it is my go-to essence whenever I feel disconnected from the grace of the natural world.

Green Nicotiana helps us to appreciate the grass that muscles its way up through concrete, and the humble whisperings of the urban trees, holding their ground and doing God's work. We notice that the empty lot next to an abandoned building that we walked past is very alive with lots of plants minding their business and doing their own thing. Green Nicotiana helps us explore how to build a functional, loving relationship with nature. It also helps us to experience and witness the resilience of nature as our hearts beat within that pulse of life. Nicotiana offers a softness of the soul as we breathe in the etheric energies of the earth. This support helps us take the edge off in the most benevolent way.

Manzanita: Get Grounded—Next we come to Manzanita flower essence, which translates from Spanish to mean "little apple tree." Manzanita is a bell-shaped flower, which in the flower essence world signifies a close relationship with the earth.[84] Manzanita is the flower essence that helps us to recognize our body as a sacred temple of spirit.

Food is one of the primary ways we nourish ourselves. The meridians of the Earth element connect to the Spleen and Stomach. Our dietary choices

---

84. "Twelve Windows of Plant Perception," Flower Society website, flowersociety.org/twelve.htm.

reflect how we nurture ourselves as well as our capacity to be nurtured by what we consume. Often someone using Manzanita flower essence will organically make dietary changes that are beneficial to them. I've had patients who have always wanted to become vegetarian. While working with Manzanita, the dietary change happens effortlessly because they have the insight and awareness of how to make it happen. On the other side of the spectrum, my vegan patients might have a Manzanita-inspired realization that they need to integrate meat into their diet. Flower essences are not interested in the cultural, political, or social dogma we humans have—they are simply concerned with what will bring us wholeness and balance. Manzanita helps us align our lifestyle with the cycles and rhythms of the earth, including our sleep and exercise habits. This flower essence sparks a desire for fresh air and helps us regulate our circadian rhythm so that we can rise and rest with the sun. Through Manzanita, we begin to worship our bodies as temples for the soul.

In my clinical practice, I have noticed that Manzanita also tends to open financial opportunities as well. The Earth element is concerned with the physical, manifested world, and our financial resources are certainly part of that. As we harmonize our relationship with the physical plane, we experience an increased capacity to attract and manage physical resources.

Manzanita helps us to fully ground into our physical bodies. When our work or lifestyle requires us to rely primarily on our intellect, this earthy essence reminds us to bring our awareness all the way down to the tips of our toes and the ground beneath our feet. If your lifestyle is very cerebral or you've experienced a trauma that makes it painful to be in different parts of your body, Manzanita is the flower essence that will support full, conscious embodiment. This flower essence is an ally for anyone who feels ungrounded or disassociated, or desires to reconnect to the vital life forces of the earth.

Embodied Practice: Parivrtta Anjaneyasana (Low Lunge Knee on Floor Pose)

Affirmation: My body is the temple for my soul.

Come into a runner's lunge position with your left foot forward between your hands. Lower your right knee to the floor. If this feels uncomfortable, place a folded blanket or pillow under your knee. Align your left knee over your left ankle. Sink your hips toward the ground to deepen the stretch.

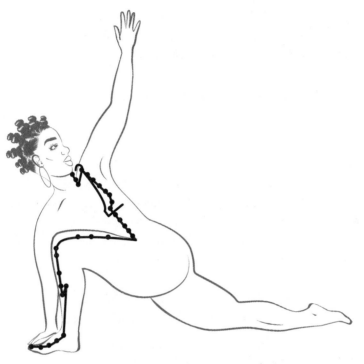

Pictured with the Stomach Meridian

While keeping your right hand on the ground alongside your left foot, gently twist at the waist to raise your left hand toward the sky. With your breath, expand through your chest as your arms form a vertical pole from the sky to the earth. Envision a stream of bright light descending from the heavens, and down into the soil.

Turn your gaze up toward your left hand to receive inspiration, or down toward your right hand to ground your vision. Recite the affirmation: *My body is a temple for my soul.*

Repeat on the opposite side.

Music Is Medicine: Playlist For the Earth Element

Earth element music helps us to feel gratitude and a sense of community within the human family. Below are some of my favorites, which all express the archetypal signatures and sounds of the Earth element.

"I Am Grateful" by Greg Stamper and Soul 21
Written/Composed by Greg Stamper © Soul21 Music (ASCAP), 2016

The Celebration Spiritual Center (CSC) in Brooklyn embodies the spirit of the Earth element. In this non-denominational church, sermons include insights from ancient and modern scripture from every culture. Pastor Greg's ad-lib reminds us that when "gratitude goes up, the miracles come down, when gratitude goes up, there's blessings all around."[85] "I Am Grateful" stirs the heart with a gratitude that resonates so strongly, your heart can't help but feel the communal abundance of the Earth element.

"Harvest for the World" by the Isley Brothers
Album: The Record Plant, T-Neck Records, 1976

The harvest of late summer is the season of the Earth element. Harvest for the World reminds us that we share our human struggles as well as our human triumphs, and collectively reap what we sow. The Earth element also teaches us that wealth, abundance, and prosperity are not for the privileged few, but for all of us.

"Kind & Generous" by Natalie Merchant
Album: Ophelia, Elektra Records 1998

The lullaby-like voice of Natalie Merchant makes this song very resonant with the Earth element. In addition to the distinct singing quality of her voice, the song evokes the Caretaker archetype. The Earth element teaches us how to extend kindness and generosity to those we love and care about, and also to ourselves.

---

85. Lyrics by Greg Stamper, Used with artist's permission.

"Lean on Me" featuring Jussie Smollett and Yazz
Album: Empire Season Five, Hollywood Records, 2020

"Lean on Me" is a remake of the song originally sung by Club Nouveau. I grew up watching the movie with the same name, about a community of young people united under the leadership of legendary principal Joe Clark. In this updated soundtrack, the cast of *Empire* comes together to remind each other that we are not in this world alone. The Earth element teaches us how to depend on one another for support and solidarity.

"Mi Gente" by J Balvin and Willy William featuring Beyoncé
Album: Vibras, Scorpio/Universal Latin, 2017

"Mi Gente" is a call for the people around the world to come together, unified by the rhythm of the music and head nod. The Earth element unifies the people, just like this trilingual dance anthem. When Beyoncé joined the remix, she announced that proceeds of the song would be donated to support disaster relief efforts in Mexico, Puerto Rico, and the Caribbean islands.[86] This compassion and willingness to support our human family would make the Earth element proud!

"Madness" by Alannis Morissette
Album: Flavors of Entanglement, Maverick/Warner Brothers, 2008

This song has a haunting eeriness but is still one of my favorites as a tribute to sympathetic resonance. The Earth element reminds us that when one heart string is plucked, the heart string of another person also vibrates. In "Madness," we see how we trigger each other's wounds as easily as we trigger each other's joy. The Earth element does not discriminate. We can resonate with any feeling, thought, or vibe in the shared human field.

---

86. Susan Cheng, "Apparently, Beyoncé Did the 'Mi Gente' Remix Because of Blue Ivy," BuzzFeed News, October 10, 2017, https://www.buzzfeednews.com/article/susancheng/beyonce-mi-gente-remix.

"We Got Love" by Teyana Taylor featuring Ms. Lauryn Hill
Album: The Album, GOOD/Def Jam Recordings, 2020

This family anthem celebrates the bonds that connect us and the love that flows through all our hearts. The Earth element helps us to cultivate gratitude for our family and community, and imagine love as the currency for abundance.

"Sing a Song" by Earth, Wind & Fire
Album: Gratitude, Columbia Records, 1975

If my life were a movie, "Sing a Song" would be the background of the opening montage of me going about my daily grind with occasional mishaps and lots of blessings. I consider it a contemporary remake of the seven dwarves' "Whistle While You Work." The Earth element reminds us to stay the course and commit to the path. When times get hard, we can sing to lift our spirits and remind ourselves of the good to come.

"Will You Be There?" by Michael Jackson
Album: Dangerous, Epic Records, 1993

The circular chorus and melody of the song brings us back around to central questions: How do we lean on each other, how do we depend on each other, and how do we support one another as a human family? The compassion of the Earth element inspires us to put aside our differences and show up for one another in our times of need.

"My Love" by Wale featuring Major Lazer, Wizkid and Dua Lipa
Album: Shine, Every Blue Moon/Maybach Music/Atlantic, 2017

The winding rhythm and melody of this song channels Earth element vibes. The Earth element is also about devotion, and our ability to hang in there 'til the end. This song champions the kind of ride-or-die commitment the Earth element inspires.

"Waiting on the World to Change" by John Mayer
Album: **Continuum,** *Aware/Sony/Columbia Records, 2006*

When we're stuck in the Earth element's spinning, we also get stuck in pro-crastination that keeps us from stepping into our power and our agency. This song describes the sluggish Earth element of a generation sitting on the side-lines, waiting to play their part to change the world.

"Hopelessly Devoted to You" by Olivia Newton John
Album: **Grease:** *The Original Soundtrack from the Motion Picture,* *RSO records, 1978*

This syrupy song can best be described as sweet and sticky, just like the Earth element. Devotion is necessary to make relationships work, but being hope-lessly devoted is another story entirely. When we find ourselves clinging to dysfunctional relationship dynamics, the Earth element helps us reconnect to our own energetic center.

"Step by Step" by Whitney Houston
Album: **The Preacher's Wife:** *Original Motion Picture Soundtrack,* *Arista/BMG Entertainment, 1996*

The Earth element reminds us to be practical. After all, Rome wasn't built in a day—someone had to carry all those bricks, one brick at a time. There is a proverb in Yorùbá that says, "Bit by bit, we eat the head of the fish," a reminder every success happens little by little. Through the Earth element, we recommit to the long haul and the load. We learn that even great works began with a single step.

"Devotion" by Earth, Wind & Fire
Album: **Open Our Eyes,** *Columbia Records, 1974*

Devotion evokes the archetypes of the Earth element as a shout out to the mothers, teachers, and caretakers of the world. The song praises the devotion that blesses children and brings light during hard times. Similarly, the Earth element teaches us that over time through devotion, we reap the fruits of our labors.

"Mama's Hand" by Queen Naija
Self-titled EP, Capitol Records, 2018

This sweet, nurturing song makes my ovaries do the wop! In the song, Queen Naija reminds her young one that no matter what he may experience, she will be there with love and devotion. When I hear this young mama speak with such tenderness and love to her cherublike toddler, it evokes the kindness, compassion, and nurturing of the Earth element.

Earth in Practice: Create a Wellness Plan

Today there are more and more resources available—Eastern, African, and Western—that teach us how to be physically healthy. We know everything there is to know, and what we don't know we can easily find online. We have endless amounts of information about our body type and the different dietary regimens. Websites like WebMD allow us to match our symptoms with illnesses so that we arrive at our doctors' offices fully informed. Our smartwatches report to us how much exercise we're getting and how much sleep we need. Yet, in the midst of this apparent health, our souls are aching.

We know that health is not just physical—it's emotional, mental, and spiritual as well. We believe there's more to life than just financial success. Our definition of health includes healthy relationships, feeling creative, living with purpose, and a sense of belonging.

Use your understanding of the subtle body and soul to create a holistic mental, emotional, and spiritual wellness regimen. Below are a few suggested modalities; make sure to include at least one healing resource for each level of your subtle body.

The Physical Body: Matter Matters

The physical body is perceived by our beta state of awareness, which is awake, responsive, and logical. Choose one of the modalities below to support your physical body (and don't forget to schedule your appointments!).

- Diet/nutrition
- Sleep hygiene (establishing a routine and environment that allows you to get the appropriate hours of sleep for your age)
- Exercise

+ Physical therapy
+ Massage
+ Finance or investment coaching (remember, the physical body includes abundance and prosperity)
+ Goal-oriented life coaching
+ Appointments with your medical providers (primary care physician, OB-GYN, etc.)
+ Prescription medications

The Etheric Body: Everything Is Energy

The etheric body is accessed by our alpha state of awareness, which is contemplative, energetic, and emotional. Choose one of the modalities below to move your qi and support your etheric body:

+ Time in nature
+ Acupuncture
+ Dance/yoga/creative movement
+ Breath work
+ Music
+ Art
+ Plant-based supplements such as essential oils, herbal supplements, and low-dose homeopathic remedies
+ Gemstone or crystal therapy
+ Reiki

The Astral Body: Change the Narrative

The astral body is accessed through our theta state of awareness, which is associative, dreamlike, and symbolic. Choose one of the modalities help you gain insight, shift your perspective, and change the narrative of your experience.

+ Flower essences
+ Journaling
+ Dreamwork
+ Individual or group therapy
+ Talking with a trusted friend

+ Social media hygiene (setting appropriate limits on your access to the thoughts and perspectives of others)
+ Astrology
+ Divination or a spiritual reading
+ Work with affirmations
+ Family Constellation healing circle

The Spiritual Body: All Is One

The spiritual body is accessed through our delta state of awareness, in addition to any tools in our spiritual practice that connect us to the Divine. Below are a few suggestions. Of course, please choose anything from your spiritual or religious practice that helps you connect to your source.

+ Reading and study of sacred texts
+ Prayer
+ Meditation
+ Chanting
+ Ritual
+ Work with archetypal energies
+ Altar building
+ Ancestor reverence

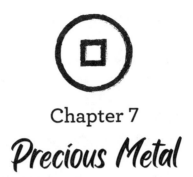

Chapter 7
Precious Metal

Throughout history, spirituality has been dedicated to the mystery of the Metal element. What happens to transform us from one experience, one reality, and one existence to the next? Metal helps us answer this question and is present in any experience that calls us to recognize the workings of a higher power. Metal is the bridge between temporal experience and the return to the Divine.

Metal Element Signatures

We recognize the archetypal qualities of the Metal element through the following signatures:

- Season: Autumn
- Phase: Completion and return
- Color: White
- Energetic: Dissipates/Dissolves qi
- Core Emotion: Grief
- Sound: Sighing/Weeping
- Meridians: Lung and Large Intestine

Season: Autumn

Autumn is my favorite season, and not just because I was born in November! Fall brings cool, crisp air and clear blue skies. In the northeastern United States, the humidity of the late summer season dissipates, allowing us to take deep, precious breaths. There's a scent in the air that reminds me of pumpkin lattes, hayrides, football, chicken wings, and spiced red wine. The leaves on trees turn breathtaking shades of gold, orange and red—a final blaze of glory before their death and descent to the earth. In a season peppered with holidays in various spiritual traditions that acknowledge the deceased and the thin veil between the physical and spiritual worlds, the Metal element also evokes nostalgia and longing for people and experiences of the past.

Phase: Completion and Return

We witness the journey through all the elements through the seasons in nature. In winter, Water gives us the seed, with destiny compressed into a promising seed of life; the acorn holding the full potential of the oak it will become. In spring, the Wood element emerges as the seed becomes a spout. In summer, we witness Fire's blossoming, flowering our landscape. In late summer, the Earth element offers abundance through fruits and harvest. The unharvested fruits fall to the earth in preparation for autumn. But then what? What happens that transforms a rotten apple fallen on the ground into the sprout that appears in spring?

The Metal element governs this invisible process of completion and return, also known as death. I consider Metal the High Priest/ess of alchemy: it transforms everything that dies into new life. This element discerns what gets composted and what gets nurtured as a seed of new energetic potential. The Metal element serves the same function in our experience and psyche, inviting us to question: Is it really junk, or something that just needs to be polished so that it can shine again? It's a question as valid for a disappointing relationship as it is for the old silverware that you found in the basement.

Think about the last major difficulty or adversity you had to face. Much of the process may have been internal. Like the rotten apple underground, you and others couldn't see the transformation happening until a new sprout emerged from the depths. Metal is the element of alchemical transformation—it transforms lead into gold, it grows the lotus from the mud, and it births the majestic scarab beetle from a ball of shit.

Metal is also present whenever we need to release something from our lives. Sometimes this is intentional—we call on Metal when we fast from unhealthy foods, habits, thoughts, and people. Sometimes Metal catches us off guard, when something or someone is taken from us by forces outside of our control. Metal affords reverence for all that is temporal, and all that is eternal. It reminds us of the inherent preciousness of our lives.

Color: White

The color associated with Metal is white. It is the natural color of chalk used to outline an ancestor shrine in Ifa culture, the bones of our body, and the ashes left behind after a fire has burned out. These aspects of white resonate with the Metal element's association with death, but also a spirit devoid of the "color" of our experiences.

Energetic: Dissolving/Dissipating

Think about the last time you had a good, hard, snot-inducing cry. That's how the qi of Metal moves. It makes hardened things soften and become less … material, less of this physical world, so to speak. Remember that apple that fell to the ground and started to compost? If we could watch the Metal element in action, we would see that apple becoming less and less of an apple, softening and dissipating until it was part of the soil from which it came. Ashes to ashes, dust to dust.

Core Emotion: Grief

It's no coincidence that grief is the emotion associated with the Metal element. Grief is the emotion we experience when we have to let go of something that had meaning and value in our lives. The Metal element encompasses the entire spectrum of grief, from deep loss to a vague sense of disappointment.

Like anger, grief is one of those emotions that can be difficult to recognize or process. We are taught at a young age that the most important thing to do with our sadness is to talk ourselves or others out of it. When we see someone crying, we almost impulsively look for something to say to make them feel better. This includes pointing out the bright side, sharing why things "aren't so bad," or jumping in with explanations of why things have to be the way they are. When these options fail us, we say things like, "try not to be sad," which is like telling a tsunami to sink quietly back into the ocean. We default to all kinds of wacky behavior to avoid our feelings of grief and to protect those around us who will feel sad if they see us grieving. We put on a brave smile to mask our pain and to keep our sadness from being contagious. Grief can also disguise itself as anger, bitterness, apathy, and hyper-rationalization as we try to avoid being overwhelmed by grief's powerful waves.

We often associate grief with death or extreme loss, but grief can show up in many ways, as often as any of the other emotions. The Metal element reminds us that grief is the appropriate emotion anytime we lose something precious. In addition to people, we can grieve the loss of intangibles like our faith, trust, hope, or time. We can grieve things that are right in front of us. We can grieve a change in our relationships, identity, routine, or lifestyle— even when it's a change for the better. Sometimes we fear that our expression of grief negates the gratitude we feel for our blessings. Yes, y'all—we can even be grieving when things are good.

I started the program in the *Grief Recovery Handbook* as I navigated grief and conflicting feelings during my daughter's transition into her teenage years. I loved who she was becoming, but how my heart ached for the little girl who greeted me with big hugs and trusted my opinion. In the handbook, I was relieved to see a list of experiences besides death and divorce—many of which are positive life events—as sources of grief:

- Moving
- Starting school
- Marriage
- Graduation
- End of addictions
- Major health changes
- Retirement
- Financial changes (positive or negative)
- Holidays
- Legal problems[87]

During the COVID pandemic, I experienced the incredible blessing of being able to transition my work into more teaching, writing, and medicine making. At the same time, I also deeply grieved the closure of my acupuncture practice, the ability to greet people with hugs, and seeing my family whenever

---

87. James John W. Friedman Russell, *The Grief Recovery Handbook: 20th Anniversary Edition: The Action Program for Moving Beyond Death, Divorce, and Other Losses* (New York: HarperCollins, 2009), 4.

I wanted to. These were all things I had taken for granted. Grief experts James and Friedman write extensively about how difficult is to deal with grief. They remind us: "grief is normal and natural, but we have been ill prepared to deal with it. *Grief is about a broken heart, not a broken brain.*"[88] The Metal element teaches us that without loss or grief, we would never learn how to honor that which is precious, valuable and sacred. Metal allows us to use grief as a bridge between that which has died, and what lives on forever in the form of memory, love, and spirit.

Below is a list of common emotions that direct us to soul medicine for the Metal element:

Reverence	Grief
Sadness	Disappointment
Despair	Nostalgia
Homesickness	Longing
Guilt	Shame
Unworthiness	

Sound: Sighing/Weeping

The sound of the Metal element in a person's voice is "sighing" or "weeping," both sounds which carry a sense of longing, breathiness, and spaciousness. We can hear a Metal quality in our voices as we recall a favorite memory, take in a deep breath, and whisper, "I miss those days" as we exhale. In music, the Metal element is present in any song that evokes a sense of wonder, grandeur and reverence. Regardless of religious affiliation, the reverence of Metal can equally be experienced with gospel music and chanting *Ohm.* Songs with flutes and other wind instruments are Metal in nature, as are songs whose lyrics convey deep longing or grief.

---

88. Friedman Russel, *Grief Recovery Handbook*, 5.

Meridians: Lung and Large Intestine

In Five Element theory, the Lungs and the Large Intestine are the organ systems of the Metal element, and they are paired for a reason. The lungs support us as we breathe in life, energy, and inspiration. And through the large intestine, we let go of what we no longer need. Skin, the largest organ of the body, is also associated with the Metal element. The skin is the boundary between ourselves and our environment.

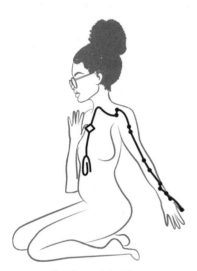

7.1 Lung Meridian

The Lung Meridian [**Figure 7.1**] starts in the lower abdomen, rises through the chest, penetrates the lungs, and travels down the arm to end at the tip of the pointer finger. The Large Intestine Meridian [**Figure 7.2**] begins at the tip of the index finger, travels along the arm, and crosses the shoulder to the back of the neck. It then continues along the side of the neck and jaw to cross the lips and end just beneath the nose.

When the Metal element meridians are compromised, some of the physical symptoms we experience include:

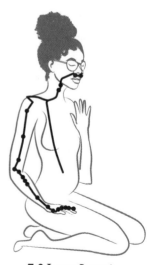

+ Skin rashes
+ Seasonal allergies (especially those that flare in autumn or spring)
+ Common cold symptoms (coughing, sneezing, stuffy head)
+ Mucus
+ Asthma
+ Bronchitis
+ Fatigue
+ Constipation
+ Shortness of breath
+ Desire to smoke

7.2 Large Intestine Meridian

We exercise the Metal element with any activity that allows us to focus on the breath. Because the lungs are neighbors to the heart, the Metal element also benefits from any cardiovascular exercise that moves qi in the chest. Swimming, running, and brisk walking are all great options. Saunas and steam rooms are also great ways to support the body in releasing toxins through the skin. When we cleanse or fast, Metal can help us process the thoughts and emotions that get stirred along with the physical release.

Soul Lesson 1: Be Present

Awaken to the mystery of being here,
and enter the quiet immensity of your own presence.
—*John O'Donohue*

Several years ago, I completed the last weekend retreat of my training in Alchemical Healing. The weekend had special significance for me—I had begun the training a year ago on my birthday weekend, so it marked the completion of a cycle, a full year of in-depth study of the five elements, the psyche, spirituality, and the unfolding of Tao in my life. A full year of growth, change, and bonding with my fellow alchemists.

I dreaded the weekend, because I do not generally do well with goodbyes; I actually avoid them. Plus, I was not quite ready to let go of the magic of the experience and wanted these spiritually immersive weekends to continue forever. I braced myself for what I expected to be a "weepy weekend." Because the training was centered on the Metal element, I was fully prepared to experience the fullness of my grief.

During the retreat, we were introduced to the *gassho rei* practice of bowing. This practice involves making eye contact, embracing, and then bowing to one another. We circled the room, bowing to each of the twenty members of the group. My eyes watered as memories surfaced from our time together. But instead of feeling sadness and grief, I felt profoundly *inspired*. I had an opportunity to acknowledge each person for their impact on my life and thank them for sharing their precious light with me. I felt a sense of completion. I was surprised to find that instead of Metal's grief, I experienced Metal's reverence and honor.

Metal teaches us how to honor our experiences in real time. We discover that even this moment—as I am writing or you are reading—has its beauty and wonder.

Reflection Questions

Are you in the here and now? Take a moment to reflect on the following questions in your journal:

- What do you do to find stillness? What gets in the way?
- What spiritual resources are supporting you?
- What worries about the past, or fears for the future, are disrupting your inner peace?
- What in your life is moving too slowly, or too quickly?
- What inspires you?

Flower Essences for Present Presence

The following flower essences support our ability to give our full attention to the present moment:

- Star Tulip to cultivate a meditative presence
- California Valerian to calm anxiety
- White Chestnut to quiet the mind
- Impatiens to support patience for process

Star Tulip: Meditative Presence—Star Tulip helps us open to a softer, more subtle and spiritual side of ourselves. Like a tree preparing for winter, Star Tulip brings our attention inward. The flower essence connects us to the secrets of the universe, and inspires us to create space for the unfolding of the great mystery.

Star Tulip is also known as cat's ears because of its soft, triangular, furry petals. These tiny antennas allow us to be receptive to experiences beyond our physical senses. Our ability to remember our dreams, hear our inner knowing, feel moved deeply, and be deeply introspective are all part of Star Tulip's wisdom.

In a modern context, Star Tulip flower essence helps us "stop and smell the roses." In our hectic and busy lives, we walk down the street with our eyes on our phone and our minds on our to-do list. Star Tulip slows us down, opening us to the subtle energies around us. Suddenly the monotony of our daily grind is infused with spirit. With Star Tulip, I stop writing to appreciate how the sunlight is shining interesting shapes on the floor of my apartment. I catch the spark in my daughter's eyes just before she delivers the punchline to one of her wacky jokes. I put down my phone for a moment to catch the breeze. This kind of noticing requires that we slow down, come out of our heads, and see the world around us through the eyes of our heart.

Star Tulip will inspire us to build an ancestral altar, start journaling or meditation practice, or seek out a religious practice or community. When my patients are working with Star Tulip , they often create a serene space in their home or office dedicated to their inner work and spirituality. Star Tulip helps us care about our inner world and experience our lives with wonder and reverence. We remember that we are indeed spiritual beings having a human experience.

Star Tulip is soul medicine for cultivating a meditative presence as we move through our day. It allows us to connect to and prioritize our spiritual life. Star Tulip serves the Metal element by helping us breathe in the sacredness of each moment and honoring the moments that take our breath away.

California Valerian and White Chestnut: Quiet the Mind and Calm Anxiety—Both California Valerian and White Chestnut blossom in clusters of small white flowers. When I gaze at the images of these flowers, I envision each blossom as a new thought or idea. And wow—is it ever noisy in there! That excessive mental activity very easily crosses over into anxiety and worry. These are exactly the conditions that California Valerian and White Chestnut help ease.

I affectionately call White Chestnut the "monkey mind flower essence," because it helps our minds to let go of the thoughts that are on constant repeat, like a broken record with a scratch. We can call on White Chestnut flower essence when we have thoughts that are repetitively circling in our heads, without any resolution or action. We mentally replay events or conversations over and over again. We find ourselves thinking: "I should have said this...", "If only I had done that ...", or "I wonder what they meant when they said _____ ," and so on (and on and on).

Most of the time, we don't even realize how busy and overactive our minds are. Mental chatter is white noise, like constant static in the background of whatever else we're trying to do. These busy thoughts keep us up at night as we stare at the ceiling, wondering if we'll ever be able to sleep.

White Chestnut also supports us when we are trying to figure something out in a very linear and logical way. Have you ever felt like your head was exploding trying to find a solution? Ever had a headache from thinking too hard? Ever squinch up your entire face as if somehow touching your nose to your forehead would activate an answer? White Chestnut is your friend. This flower essence quiets the mind and welcomes inner spaciousness in our thinking processes. It may bring new awareness to the worries in heavy rotation, so that we can take action or make the necessary changes in our lives to quiet them. White Chestnut can also help us value not knowing or having an answer, as well as being in the moment so that we can hear our intuition with more clarity.

Like White Chestnut, California Valerian flower essence also helps to quiet an overactive mind. In herbal medicine, valerian root is a popular nervine and sedative for the nervous system. California Valerian as a flower essence has a similarly calming effect—it settles excessive negative thoughts and worries about the future. We can call on California Valerian when we create worst-case scenarios in our mind. Our mental static is filled with thoughts such as *If I do this, then xyz will happen* or *If I don't do xyz, then abc won't happen.* It's a mental trap that takes us out of the here and now and eclipses our appreciation of the present moment.

Here's a transcription of a common inner monologue:

I don't make enough money. If I don't make enough money ... then I won't be able to pay my rent. If I don't pay my rent ... we will get evicted. If we get evicted.... Then my daughter and I will be homeless. If my daughter and I are homeless ... I will fail as a parent.

Okay, so maybe this not a common train of thought; maybe it's just *my* inner dialogue. And as I write it, I see it's totally ridiculous. I can see that when I am caught in a whirlwind of anxiety about my finances, I bypass my creative money instincts. I'm ignoring that I have tons of friends and family who would take me in if I fell on hard times. I'm ignoring that it's my love, time, and emotional presence that make the biggest impact on my parenting. I'm unable to see that abundance is everywhere, and that I am actually quite blessed to have a career that I love. The point is, my monkey mind is totally disconnected from my higher self, the part of me that sees clearly and intuits solutions.

White Chestnut and California Valerian are often the first flower essences I consider for patients who have a hard time quieting their minds for meditation or shutting off their to-do list while on the acupuncture table. Just like a snow globe, these sister flowers settle the flurries of our thoughts so that we can calmly perceive the present moment without worry or anxiety. I love hearing my patients express, "I have way more time than I used to now that I'm not always thinking!"

Impatiens: Patience for Process—Like California Valerian, when we need Impatiens flower essence, we are often mentally living two or three steps in the future! This flower is named for the way its seeds explode from their pods when touched, spewing their seeds several meters away. In the same way, the person needing Impatiens may explode when provoked. Road rage, Monday morning meetings without coffee, kids who don't respect bedtime, and people doing generally dumb stuff are all situations in which Impatiens could certainly work some magic. Maybe one day it will rain down from the heavens and make New York a nicer place.

Impatiens is one of the flower essences indicated for irritability, which it certainly addresses. But on a deeper level, Impatiens addresses soul agitation that stems from wanting things to be different than they actually are. When we are in an Impatiens state, we want people around us to change. We want others to hurry up and move more quickly. Or we want something in our life to be over and done with already! It doesn't matter if we're talking about an argument, a financial downfall, a legal battle, or the line at the post office.

Our impatience can even be directed at our own growth or healing and periods that require the slow, intentional process of inner transformation. I've given Impatiens to clients who were ready to throw in the towel with dating, and those ready to send their wayward kids off to boarding school. Impatiens supported another client through her recovery from abdominal surgery, balancing her desire to resume exercise with the time her body needed to heal. Impatiens can even be an ally in labor and delivery, for women who are having a difficult time staying present in the process.[89]

---

89. Please consult a trained flower essence practitioner or doula before using flower essences during pregnancy or labor.

Impatiens is the soul medicine of choice when we are specifically agitated by the pace of people or a process. It is equally relevant for that person who's frustrated with the timing of their career as it is for that parent who wants their child to move faster in the morning to get ready for school. It is useful in relationships where there is conflict, especially when one person wants the other to make immediate changes. Impatiens may bring awareness to an unconscious inner dialogue in which we are constantly asking, *"Why don't you get it fast enough?" "Why aren't things changing fast enough?" "Why aren't things the way they are in my mind?"* Impatiens gifts us with the miracle of patience for process, easing us into the awareness we can only be right here, right now. It teaches us that this very moment deserves our full and complete attention.

Embodied Practice: Tadasana (Mountain Pose)

Affirmation: I am here, now.

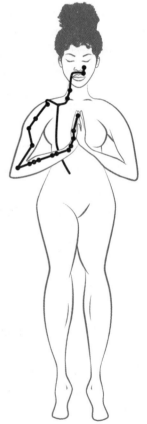

Stand with your feet firmly rooted into the ground. Press your hands together in prayer position. Roll your shoulders back and down, and imagine the top of your head reaching toward the sky, finding length in your back and neck. Take several deep breaths at your own pace to ground yourself into the present moment.

With a soft gaze, bring your attention to the first color you see. Then slowly gaze around the room, mentally naming everything you see that is a variation of that color. Repeat several times, using different colors as your starting point, until you feel a calm awareness of your environment.

Close with the affirmation: *I am here, now.*

**Pictured with the
Large Intestine Meridian**

Soul Lesson 2:
You Are Precious

We ask ourselves, who am I to be brilliant, gorgeous, tatented, fabulous?
Actually, who are you not to be?
—Marianne Williamson

The Metal element teaches us how to discern the extraordinary from the ordinary. It discovers the divine within the mundane. The metaphor for this hidden mystery is described in many spiritual traditions: in East Asian spirituality as a beautiful lotus flower emerges from the mud. In the Kemetic tradition, the exquisite Khepri beetle is born in a ball of dung. In the Christian tradition, water is transformed into wine. Metal governs alchemy, the science of transformation. Soul alchemy transforms the lead of our lives—the difficult, challenged, or stuck places—into gold: the illuminated qualities of insight, awareness, love, and joy. Metal teaches us that the spirit of the divine is within every aspect of earthly substance and earthly experience.

Imagine you are a gold miner in the early nineteenth century. Knee-deep in mud, you use your pan to sort through all the muck. If you're lucky, you catch a shimmer peeking out from beneath a mud-covered rock. In most cases, you'd bypass the precious metal, throwing it out with the rocks. And just like early nineteenth-century gold miners, we can become obsessed with finding something precious and valuable—like gold—in ourselves and each other. We know it's in there somewhere, so we keep digging, looking, and seeking by demanding perfection or setting impossibly high standards. While sifting through the mud and dirt, we throw away the gold that is right in front of us.

The Metal element helps us to see preciousness first in ourselves and then in those around us. It restores the integrity of our radiant, inner divinity, and invites us to experience radical self-love. Metal gifts us with the ability to witness, acknowledge, and honor our inner light. We bow to each other in the spirit of the Hindu greeting *namaste*, which translates as "the divine in me salutes and honors the divine in you."

When we are disconnected from Metal's gift of positive self-regard, we experience a sense of inadequacy.[90] We might seek praise and validation from others to override our internal low-esteem. We may overwork or rely on material status symbols of our success. When Metal is out of balance, things are never quite enough: our house is never quite clean enough, our work is never quite good enough, our relationships are never quite loving enough. We may attempt to control others, mistakenly believing that perfect order reflects our perfect selves. Metal then becomes brittle and cold, and can make us distant, aloof, hypercritical, or abrasive. This stance in the world may protect us from feeling vulnerability and shame, but it also disconnects us from our spiritual radiance. The Metal element helps to cultivate an inner sense of preciousness to counter these defenses.

Disconnection from our inner gold can also make us over-apologetic and self-effacing. We may lack the confidence to negotiate for our value in the world. We may feel inferior to our peers and colleagues. On a spiritual level, the Metal element can help us to experience the greatness of ourselves, fueling us with the courage to take a stand for what we deserve.

Finally, the Metal element helps us find forgiveness for our flaws and acceptance of our imperfections. With Metal, we move through the shame, self-doubt, and criticism we put on ourselves. We find the signature of a healthy Metal element in a person whose power seems to come from beyond the physical world. In the presence of healthy Metal, we sit up a bit straighter. An air of royalty evokes respect, esteem and honor. The Metal element helps us experience ourselves as royal and divine.

Reflection Questions

Take a moment to consider your greatness, and then reflect on the following questions in your journal:

+ What do you love about your body, your mind, and your heart?
+ When are you most comfortable in your own skin?

---

90. Angela Hicks, John Hicks, and Peter Mole, *Five Element Constitutional Acupuncture* (Edinburgh, UK: Churchill Livingstone, 2011), 143–149.

+ What are you proud of?
+ What makes you unique?
+ Who are the people in your life who encourage, motivate, and celebrate you?
+ What influences send the message that you are not good enough?

Flower Essences for Increasing Our Self-Worth

The following flower essences help us to cultivate radical self-love and positive self-esteem

+ Gold essence to know our worth
+ Buttercup for humble radiance
+ Pink Monkeyflower for confident vulnerability
+ Pine for self-acceptance

Gold: Know Your Worth—In the book *Money Is Love: Connecting to the Sacred Origins of Money*, Barbara Wilder discusses the first currencies that emerged during the Iron Age, gold and silver, as representatives of the sacred energies of the sun and moon. She writes:

> To understand this concept, imagine yourself as a member of a Neolithic village. Everything in your life depends on the reaping of a good harvest. The sun must shine on the crops all summer long to ensure a good harvest. The god who is the sun must be worshipped and revered to ensure a good harvest. Recently, gold has been discovered and you, knowing that all things in the heavens and on earth are on one great cosmic dance, now hold a piece of gold in your hands. To you, this is not an inanimate object that shines and reflects the sun's light. This is a piece of the divine sun itself. And the fact that you are holding a piece of God in your hand means that you have a sacred responsibility.[91]

91. Barbara Wilder, *Money Is Love: Reconnecting to the Sacred Origins of Money* (London: Cygnus Books, 2010), 27.

Gold is represented in the periodic table of elements is (Au), at the root of words such as *aurora* and *aura*, which all refer to light and radiance. Gold essence connects us to this sacred light within our soul, and to this divine responsibility. It awakens the ability to know that in the core of our being we are valuable. This value comes not from what we *do*, but from who we *are*. Gold essence affirms that we are indeed worthy of the goodness that comes our way. It awakens the valuable "gold" at the center of our being, and helps us to radiate that value into the world. Gold essence reminds us that our true value and our true worth come from our connection to this divine and royal part of ourselves.

I almost always offer Gold essence to my patients as they are entering salary negotiations for new positions or for annual bonuses. One of my patients was a mid-level executive in an arts organization in the midst of major layoffs. She had played a critical yet undervalued role keeping the organization afloat during a tough fiscal year. While working with the Gold essence, I asked her to create a list of all she that had contributed to the company in the past year. As we reviewed the list, she sat up noticeably straighter, with the proud presence that is a signature of the Metal element. I suggested that she request a promotion to a director position, with a 25K salary increase. Her eyes grew wide in disbelief at the audacity of the ask, but not as wide as they grew when she got the promotion *and* the raise!

There is lots of research out there about gender and racial inequalities in the workforce. One of my favorite resources is *Nice Girls Still Don't Get the Corner Office*, by Lois Frankel. In it, she describes four reasons for the gender inequities in salaries.[92]

1. Entitlement: Women did not feel as entitled to make more than their colleagues
2. Worth: Women felt uncomfortable measuring their worth
3. Proving Oneself: Women were less likely to use past experiences as rationale for more money

---

92. Lois Frankel, *Nice Girls Don't Get the Corner Office: Unconscious Mistakes Women Make That Sabotage Their Careers* (New York: Grand Central Publishing, 2014), 254–256.

4. Consequences: Women feared they would be perceived negatively if they asked for more money

In my practice, I've found that Gold essence helps counter all of these psychic glitches—sometimes even without understanding how or why. I've also found this essence particularly useful for entrepreneurs who undercharge for services because they've underestimated their own value!

It's important to remember that Gold is not just about financial abundance. This remedy helps us recognize that are worthy of abundance in the form of love, time, family, community, laughter, joy, and safety.

Buttercup: Humble Radiance—Buttercup flower essence reminds me of the traditional gospel song "This Little Light of Mine." Originally recorded in 1939 by John Lomax, this song is taught to children in every Baptist bible school I've ever known, The lyrics remind us repeatedly not to be afraid to let the little light of our divinity shine. Just singing that song in my head brings a gentle, warm smile to my heart. Buttercup flower essence helps us to shine our light in the world, no matter how small that light may be. Even the smallest light can cut through darkness.

Buttercup flower essence is for when we experience ourselves as inadequate. The key language that cues the need for Buttercup is "not enough." Sometimes we tell ourselves (unconsciously, of course) that we are not smart enough, trained enough, tall enough, thin enough, pretty enough, loved enough. We are not _____ enough (fill in the blank). You get the picture! The list of negative things we say to and about ourselves can be endless.

Buttercup helps us feel comfortable in our own skin and acknowledge our successes and contributions, no matter how small. It's a great flower essence for children, because children often say to themselves things such as:

- "I'm too small to be important."
- "I'm too little to do anything."
- "I'm not big enough to make a difference."
- "I'm not smart enough to pass this test."

Buttercup also has a strong resonance with the inner child in all of us looking for proof that we are, in fact, enough. I've used Buttercup for spouses who feel like they don't contribute enough to the family's income, or friends who don't feel confident enough to post on social media.

The sixty-second hexagram in the *I Ching* speaks to the modesty and power of this little light.[93] In one of the most popular translations of this ancient text used today, Richard Wilheim names this hexagram "Preponderance of the Small."[94] The hexagram describes situations where it is important to not take big, grandiose actions. Rather, success and power come from staying humble, low to the ground, and earnest in one's tasks. Buttercup helps us to acknowledge the power of our inner light, rather than making the big, external gestures in an effort to gain recognition or praise.

Buttercup invites us to the miracle of knowing that "We are enough" and that we are precious just the way we are. We don't need praise or external validation for our little lights to shine.

Pink Monkeyflower: Confident Vulnerability—Imagine that you've stepped onto center stage, prepared to sing a solo. For some of us, that image alone is enough to trigger embarrassment. Now imagine that as the curtain rises in front of an audience of your closest friends and biggest critics, you look down and notice that you forgot to get dressed. What do you do? Stand brazenly in your nakedness, completely exposed? Or run offstage and hide?

We each answer this question differently, as we each have different degrees to which we can feel comfortable being seen. Pink Monkeyflower addresses the desire to run and hide, to conceal ourselves rather than letting ourselves shine. This flower essence helps us cultivate our capacity for emotional exposure.

Whether we hide from sharing emotions in an intimate relationship, or hide our brilliance in an executive board meeting, Pink Monkeyflower flower essence addresses our capacity to be revealed. Sharing ourselves—our work, our ideas, our creativity, and our feelings—requires risk. *What if others don't love or appreciate us? What if we are criticized?* These fears can be paralyzing and create an energetic block to our fullest life. Pink Monkeyflower empowers us to fearlessly share our light, and to be vulnerable enough to reveal ourselves. How do we allow ourselves to be seen? What parts of ourselves do we

---

93. Also called the *Book of Changes*, the *I Ching* is a divination system birthed in ancient China. It consists of eight symbolic trigrams and sixty-four hexagrams that describe the alternating relationships between yin and yang.

94. Wilheim and Baynes, *The I Ching*, 127s.

conceal, and why? Pink Monkeyflower invites us to explore our answers to these questions.

In her book *Daring Greatly*, shame researcher and author Brené Brown deeply explores the relationship between shame and vulnerability. Her writing gives contemporary context and depth to the ancient relationship between Fire and Metal:

> Shame is the fear of disconnection—it's the fear that something we've done or failed to do, and ideal that we've not lived up to, or a goal that we've not accomplished makes us unworthy of connection. I'm not worthy or good enough for love, belonging or connection. I'm unlovable. I don't belong. Here's the definition of shame that emerged from my research: Shame is the intensely painful feeling that or experience of believing that we are flawed, and therefore unworthy of love and belonging.[95]

We may have received messages during childhood that instilled a sense of shame, possibly due to strict upbringing or impossibly high standards (the Metal element at its worst). Working with Pink Monkeyflower often brings our awareness to moments in the past where we felt like we didn't measure up. Whatever the cause, the fear of being criticized or rejected can make it difficult for someone needing Pink Monkeyflower to open to others. This challenge of being vulnerable or tenderly exposed directly affects the success of our most important relationships—personal and professional. Pink Monkeyflower helps us radiate *Here I am. You can see me, and I'm not afraid to shine.*

Pink Monkeyflower offers the gift of feeling safe to be seen. Whether we're sharing our feelings with a lover, sharing our art with a public audience, or taking the lead in a company, we learn that we can continue to shine and radiate while being witnessed by the world. With this inner shine in place, we feel confident while being vulnerable or exposed.

Pine: Self-acceptance—There is an old saying that says, "Be humble, for you are of the earth. Be noble, for you are of the stars." Pine flower essence

---

95. Brené Brown, *Daring Greatly: How the Courage to Be Vulnerable Transforms the Way We Live, Love, Parent, and Lead* (New York: Penguin Random House Audio Publishing Group, 2017), 68–71.

is an ally when our attachment to the earth, to the fallible, human side of us keeps us from acknowledging the divine essence of our being. It supports us when we are attached to our past transgressions, and walk with an inner checklist of all the reasons we should be deemed unworthy. Pine helps us realize that even if we make mistakes, we are perfectly imperfect. Our bad choices, the times we've put our foot in our mouths, and the opportunities we may have missed don't take away from our essential worth. Pine helps to silence self-defeating thoughts, especially if those thoughts are tied to a specific action or incident.

Like Pink Monkeyflower, Pine supports us as we move through internalized shame. Sometimes our shame is rooted in current habits, while other times it is rooted in our childhood wounds. As children, we tend to blame ourselves for everything. Our inner child organizes the world in faulty logic, creating narratives such as "My parents got divorced because I didn't go to bed on time." As adults, we can continue to create narratives that center us as the blame within circumstances that are beyond our control.

Pine facilitates an awareness of our sources of guilt or shame so that we can face them directly. If we are culpable, we are empowered to own our mistakes, apologize, and take corrective actions to make amends. We can move forward knowing that we did our best to right our wrongs, releasing the hold of the negative thoughts that haunt us. If the shame or guilt we feel rooted in something beyond our power, we are able to gain a healthy perspective, and even recognize the humanity of those who have wronged us. In this way, we reclaim our personal power and self-esteem. Other times, Pine helps us find grace and self-acceptance when we fall short of high standards and expectations, either from others or ourselves.

When out of balance, the Metal element has a tendency crystallize our faults, keeping us stuck in past mistakes. Pine helps us accept those faults as part of what makes us human. As we release guilt and shame, we find acceptance that allows us to move forward into our fullest, most expansive selves.

Embodied Practice: Urdhva Hastasana (Upward Salute)

Affirmation: I am precious.

Start in tadasana, with your hands in prayer position as your feet root into the earth. Next, extend your hands to the sky, as if offering a prayer to the sun. Envision a stream of sunlight flowing through your arms, pouring into your heart's center. Lift your chest and come into a slight backbend. Now envision that golden light radiating from your center and out into the world.

Close your eyes and repeat the affirmation: *I am precious.*

Soul Lesson 3: Let It Go

When I let go of what I am,
I become what I might be.
—Lao Tzu

Letting go is a natural part of the cycle of life. Can you imagine what would happen if we only breathed in but never exhaled? We would explode! Or if we only ate, but never took a shit, we'd also be really, really sick. In nature, there is a natural balance of receiving and releasing, inhaling and exhaling. There is a time to welcome in new opportunity, and another time to let go. The ability to take in our experiences and form relationships allows us to fully participate in life, while the ability to let go of our experiences allows us to mature with wisdom.

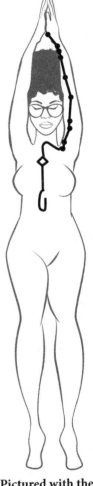

Pictured with the Lung Meridian

When something or someone has completed its time in our lives, Metal urges us to let it go. The emotion associated with this process is grief. Grief weighs us down with the "gone too soon" feeling and longing for what can no longer be. Grief also allows us to truly honor the sacredness of what we have lost. And often honoring—through prayer, ritual, art, community or even time—is the only thing that can pull us through grief. That's why Metal gifts us with the spiritual practices that fill us with reverence for our worldly experiences, and reverence for what lies beyond.

We can learn the delicate art of letting go from nature, during autumn—the season of the Metal element. In the northeast, we see leaves changing from bright reds and yellows to rusty browns. I notice as they dance joyfully in the wind before finding a resting place on the earth. The release is effortless, full of ease and grace. The tree is not pushing the leaves away. In fact, the tree is simply doing what it must at this time of year: bringing its energy, attention, life force inward to prepare for winter. It is the ultimate act of self-care and self-preservation. The tree doesn't say, "Leaves, get on out of here!" Rather, because it is no longer trying to hold on to those leaves, they are free to fly in the wind. Easy, breezy, *ahhh*.

For some reason, my "letting go" is always just the opposite—full of struggle, full of resistance, full of angst and heartache, full of long and wailing moans to my besties: "But *whyyy?*" Then the withdrawal symptoms kick in: obsessive thoughts, irritability, sadness, and denial. Good grief (Metal pun intended).

But in nature, the leaves *dance*. I imagine the spirit of the tree offering a raspy prayer of gratitude to the leaves as the wind carries them:

> *Beloved leaves: thank you so much for bringing in the sun for the past six months. Thank you for offering shade to those who rested by my side. Thank you for the life force that was once part of you, and is now part of me. Our time together has ended, and I love you for what we shared. As I withdraw and turn inward, you are free to fly.*

And then I imagine myself offering the same prayer of gratitude to the things I struggle to release from my life:

> *Dear Caramel Latte: Thank you so much for greeting me every morning. But, I am sleeping and exercising more now, so I no longer need you to feel awake and kind. I love you, but I withdraw from you and release you from my life. Plus, you make me bloated.*

> *Dear Sugar: Thank you so much for your deliciousness. I've decided to focus on new ways to fill my life with sweetness. I love you, probably always will, but I withdraw from you and release you from my life.*

(Note to self: Just because you will miss something does *not* mean it's good for you. Or that you're supposed to have it. Repeat three times and click your heels.) Which brings me to ...

*Dear Lover: Thank you for your gentle touch and for healing parts of me
I did not know needed healing. But my focus is different now. As I withdraw and turn inward, you are free to fly.*

I say this silent prayer to all of my bad habits and addictions: my work
addiction, my helicopter parenting, my curious addiction to chocolate-covered
caramel pretzels (don't judge). I acknowledge the purpose that each has served
me and realign with the integrity at the core of my being. I challenge myself to
let go without struggle with effort toward that easy-breezy feeling of autumn
leaves.

Reflection Questions

Take a deep exhale, and then reflect on the following questions in your journal:

  + What thoughts, feelings or habits are you ready to release?
  + What attachments to others are holding you back?
  + What can you let go of in your environment that is taking up too
    much space?
  + What in your diet or health regimen no longer serves you?
  + What from the past are you bringing into the present moment? How
    can you honor it, let it go, or both?
  + What is opening for you in the spaces where you let go? What are
    you welcoming in?

Flower Essences to Support an Energetic Release

The following flower essences help us to let go with grace and ease:

  + Rock Water to release rigidity and find fluidity
  + Sagebrush to clear the clutter
  + Bleeding Heart to let go with love

Rock Water: Let Go and Let Flow—We experience metal as solid and
unyielding. Metals, gemstones, diamonds, and crystals are all natural forms of
the Metal element. Yet, we also know that over time, water has power to gently
erode even the hardest rocks. Rock Water functions in a similar way, gently
eroding hardened routines and crystallized habits to create flexibility and flow.
Rock Water brings our attention to the rigid parts of ourselves. It offers grace,
allowance, and surrender so that there can be more fluidity in our experience.

Rock Water is best for releasing dogmatic ideals. It softens the hard edges of our expectations for ourselves and others. One of my favorite patients perfectly expressed the energetic of Rock Water when he shared, "I hate cold showers. But I take one every single morning for exactly thirty seconds because I know it's good for my circulation." Healthy commitment and discipline notwithstanding, a person needing Rock Water may feel guilt or shame when they are unable to meet the impossibly high or rigid standards they set for themselves.

In my practice, I know to call on Rock Water whenever I hear a patient frequently use the word "should." It's amazing how that six-letter word has the power to make us bypass our desires, personal agency, and our intuition. In her book, *SHOULD: How the Habits of Language Shape Our Lives*, Rebecca Smith warns us about how the use of the word creates a sense of obligation to what she calls the "unseen oppressor."[96] This ever-watchful eye stands guard over us, making sure we measure up to the standards society has shaped for us. Rock Water helps us look that internalized oppressor in the eye and live our lives with increased authenticity.

Rock Water also helps us release our need for control. It softens uncompromising ideas about the way we want ourselves, our lives, and others to be. A person working with Rock Water may begin to acknowledge the places where they try to exert too much control and the fears that might be suppressed. One example is having an overly strict diet due to underlying fears about gaining weight. Unprocessed fear of being abandoned or betrayed may result in us having strict demands for relationships. Or, we might have strict demands for children out of fear of being a "bad parent."

Rock Water invites us to let go and let flow, so that we may experience less tension, and more ease.

Sagebrush: Clear the Clutter—I call Sagebrush the Marie Kondo of the flower essence world. Her book, *The Life-Changing Magic of Tidying Up*, inspired millions to get rid of lots and lots of shit. She challenged us to examine what and why we have what we have and to only keep things which are meaningful and purposeful. And that's exactly what Sagebrush helps us to do.

---

96. Rebecca Smith and Marie Manthey, *Should: How Habits of Language Shape Our Lives* (Minneapolis, MN: Creative Health Care Management, 2016), 28.

I envision the dry, fingerlike leaves of this aromatic shrub as a psychic broom for whatever we want to get rid of. Sagebrush brings our awareness to people, places, situations, and unwanted perspectives that it's time to sweep away. Like its botanical relative sage, the shrub can be burned to purify and sweep out any negative energies in our physical space. Sagebrush as a flower essence has a similar action within our mental and emotional space.

Many people have heard the story of the monkey and the banana trap. If you haven't, here's a quick recap. The monkey trappers are trying to find a way to catch monkeys. So they make a special box with a banana inside. The monkeys, being the banana-lovers that they are, can't resist reaching into the small hole at the top of the box for the treat. The problem is that with their little fist clamped so tightly around the banana, they can't get their hand and the banana out of the box. They are trapped…but if they could simply let go, they would be free.

Stop here and take a minute to fill in this statement: If I could just let go of _____ , then I could be/ have _____.

The problem with the monkey trap story is that, like most of us, the monkey simply doesn't want to let go. And why should it? Sure, there could be freedom, but that's a pretty abstract concept to trade in for the ripe juicy banana right there in front of it. And if you look at your statement above, whatever you put in the second blank might be just as abstract…because it isn't here yet. This is where many of us get stuck. Sometimes we know exactly what we have to let go of. We even know why. But the thought of letting it go for the promise of something intangible often makes us hold on even more tightly. Sure, this anger, this relationship, this clutter, etc. might need to go, but without it, what guarantees do we have? It's a big mystery to wrap our monkey-minds around, one that requires trust in the Great Mystery.

Once while working with Sagebrush, I put twelve—yes, *twelve*—bags of I don't even know what in the garbage. I was obsessed with cleaning my closets and under my bed. Even more remarkably, I found myself reevaluating my relationships. I explored friendships that I needed to invest more time in, as well as those that needed a pause. My entire life got lighter, freer, and more spacious inside and out.

The realization that something doesn't serve us anymore can be painful, but it is the first step toward moving it out of our lives. I had one patient whose work with Sagebrush made her realize that her emotionally abusive marriage was broken beyond repair. Another realized it was time to start looking for a new job, one that valued her creativity and leadership skills. The latter was after nearly three months of frustration, anger, and trying to make it work.

When we try to actively push someone or something away, we end up holding on even tighter. We become stuck in the metaphorical banana trap. Sagebrush offers the miracle of effortless release by redirecting our attention and energy toward what's core, what we value, and what's essential. It helps us focus on what we *do* need instead of holding on to what we don't.

Bleeding Heart: Let Go with Love—In our chest, the lungs of the Metal element and the heart of the Fire element sit right next to each other. When we're releasing anything from our life, we also have to let it go from our heart. Grief emerges during divorce, death, and conflicts that force us to separate from someone we love. Even exciting changes—like moving to a new city or having a baby—can trigger feelings of sadness as we let go of what was familiar and comfortable.

Bleeding Heart is one of the most popular flower essences used in my practice. Have you ever seen one of those cartoon pictures of a heart with holes in it, blood leaking out everywhere? That's the kind of situation that calls for Bleeding Heart flower essence. The flower itself consists of bright pink bulbs in the shape of hearts, drooping from a vine-like branch. This flower acts as an emotional bandage for the leaking heart that is not being replenished. Often, the pain and emptiness of letting go makes us cling on even tighter.

Bleeding Heart helps us to consolidate those love forces. When we are in a relationship, we share a part of ourselves; there is a merging and blending of heart forces, just as two candles brighten when they join. Bleeding Heart addresses the pain of separation, when the two candles come apart and still shine independently. This separation shows up in many ways: a loved one dies, a bitter breakup, a friend moves to another state and can't spend Fridays on the couch with you anymore. I was in a Bleeding Heart state when my daughter turned into a teenager overnight and I missed our connection so badly that it made my heart ache.

No matter the cause, the appropriately named Bleeding Heart is a widely applicable flower essence for self-containment during separation. It helps us when we blur the boundary of where we begin and others end. It balances our ability to love fully while simultaneously connecting to a divine love within ourselves. This emotional containment and freedom allows us to truly be in choice about how we relate to others. It moves us beyond compulsive attachment, inappropriate enmeshment, and clinging desperation. It is soul medicine for the grief of a broken heart.

Bleeding Heart allows us to let go with love. It requires that we seal up those holes in our heart and keep some of the divine love inside for ourselves. Once that happens, we can send our love through any emotional, physical, or spiritual distance.

Embodied Practice: Uttanasana (Standing Forward Bend)

Affirmation: I let go, I release, I surrender.

Start in urdhva hastasana with your hands in prayer extended to the sky. Call to mind something you are ready to release. With a deep bow, bend at the hips and fold forward over your legs. Bring your hands to rest on the floor or your shins, or grab opposite elbows. If this feels uncomfortable, bend your knees slightly until you find ease.

Envision all of what you'd like to release flowing through your arms and releasing into the earth. Allow nature to receive this offering, and transmute your experience into wisdom and insight.

In your deep bow, repeat the affirmation: *I let go, I release, I surrender.*

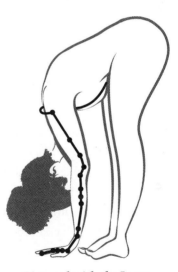

Pictured with the Large Intestine Meridian

Music Is Medicine:
Playlist For the Metal Element

A Metal element playlist is perfect for whenever you want to feel connected to Spirit, or to someone or something no longer in your life. Sometimes, Metal element songs release our tears so that we can process our grief and sadness. Metal songs also instill a deep reverence for the power of the sacred. The songs below express the archetypal sounds and signatures of the Metal element.

"Sueno Con Ella (I Dream of Her)" by Buika
Album: La noche más larga, *Warner Music Spain, 2013*

The aching, gut-wrenching wail of Buika gives voice to the profound grief and longing of the Metal element. Whether through death, divorce, or plain ol' universal experience, the pain of losing someone we cherish is undeniable. In "Sueno con Ella," the singer dreams of her beloved—reliving their experiences through the ephemeral images stored in her heart. In the same way, Metal helps us connect on a soul level to those who are no longer with us, affirming that our bond to those we've loved and lost is never truly broken.

"Growing Old/13th Floor" by OutKast
Album: ATLiens, *LaFace Records, 1996*

In typical Metal element fashion, the *ATLiens* album conjures waves of nostalgia for days gone by. The somber tonality of "Growing Old" and the lyrics of the chorus evoke the quiet, inspired stillness of Metal. It reminds us that in order for change to happen, we must first let go, and this element helps us do just that. Metal supports us in releasing what no longer serves us—negative emotions, bad habits, even clutter in the house—so that we become all we might be.

"Say Something" by A Great Big World
featuring Christina Aguilera
Album: Is There Anybody Out There?, *Epic Records, 2014*

Their performance of this song on *The Voice* with songbird Christina Aguilera brought A Great Big World onto the world stage. This song is one of the most heartbreaking I've ever heard! It opens with piano chords that remind me of autumn leaves gently surrendering to the earth, just as the lyrics represent that final moment of letting go.

"Slowly, Surely" by Jill Scott
Album: Who is Jill Scott?: Words and Sounds Vol. 1,
Hidden Beach, 2000

The whiny, melodic intro to this song before the beat drops sounds just like the wispiness of Metal element in a person's voice. When our Metal is healthy, we are able to stand in our worth and walk away from anything that doesn't honor us. Even though heartache may make clinging to the past tempting, the Metal element helps us to move forward with the grace and self-assuredness of Queen Jilly from Philly.

"Lost Ones" by Jay-Z featuring Chrissette Michelle
Album: Kingdom Come, *Roc-A-Fella Records/Def Jam Recordings, 2006*

Business partners, friends, lovers, family—everyone is in our life for a reason, season, or lifetime. And whether by choice or by circumstance, there may come a time to part ways. It's worth noting that grief does not always show up as sadness. I love this song because the dance of Metal's grief and Wood's anger in "Lost Ones" give us a different picture of how we move through loss.

"Higher" by DJ Khaled, Nipsey Hustle, and John Legend
Album: Father of Asahd,
We the Best/Epic/Roc Nation, 2019

The first time I heard this song, I immediately burst into uncontrollable tears—part of it was because the song was released in loving memory of the song's featured artist, Nipsey Hustle, a young brother gone way too soon. Another part was because the awesome power of the Metal element brings us to our knees: to weep, to pray, or both. Like the Metal element, this song calls us to lift our souls higher—in life and in death.

"More to Life" by Fertile Ground
Album: Seasons Change, *BlackOut Studios, 2000*

The Metal element gifts us with inspiration, the ability to see beyond the everyday to the quintessential divinity of all life. But sometimes in our day-to-day routine, we lose sight of that inspiration, giving rise to fatigue and the Monday morning blues…every day. When you feel the dreariness of the mundane or overwhelmingly uninspired, call on the Metal element (or this song!) to give your soul an inspired lift.

"Bigger" by Beyoncé
Album: The Lion King, Parkwood Columbia, 2019

In this ballad by Beyonce, we are reminded that we are so much bigger than we can even imagine. This spiritual song honors the Divine manifesting through us as the living word. When we feel small, unimportant, or unworthy, the Metal element brings us back to our divine essence—an essence that is connected to the entire universe. The subtle organ chords in the background take us to church, one of the places the Metal element likes to hang out.

"Angel" by Sarah McLachlan
Album: Surfacing, Nettwerk (Canada), *Arista, 1997*

The hauntingly angelic and breathless voice of Sarah McLachlan in this song is oh so Metal. Through the Metal element we find redemption and freedom from suffering as our experiences are refined and transmuted to the highest good of humanity. In our deepest moments of loneliness and despair, the Metal element helps us remember that we are never truly alone. Our ancestors and guardians stand ever ready to support—or carry—us through tough times.

"Star People" by Fertile Ground
Album: Seasons Change, *BlackOut Studios, 2000*

"Star People" is a Metal element classic. Not only does it honor the beings of light who have passed on or are getting ready to be born, it reminds us to look skyward and connect to our true purpose. The Metal element helps us listen to the subtle whispering of our souls, allowing us to slow down enough to reconnect to why we are here and what we are really up to.

"7 Years" by Lukas Graham
Album: Lukas Graham, *Copenhagen Records*, 2015

The Metal element evokes nostalgia, as does the sound of the vintage film strip in the background of this beautiful song. Lukas Graham reminisces about the most precious moments of their life as though watching a movie. In a similar way, the Metal element offers us the ability to reflect on our experiences over the span of time. Metal reminds us to spend our time making beautiful memories, because our time on Earth will at some point come to an end.

"As" by Stevie Wonder
Album: Songs in the Key of Life, *Tamia Records*, 1976

There is a side of my family that plays this joyous song at every celebration of life. At birthdays, graduations, and even funerals, we can look forward to pulling up the lyrics on our phones and singing along. "As" reminds us that our essence is love, in all ways, always. It transcends space and time—and our physical existence. Just as the heart and lungs live next to each other in our chest, our grief for what we've lost can live next to our joy of what *is*. The Metal element teaches us that our essence is eternal.

"Breathe" by Telepopmusik
Album: Genetic World, *Catalogue/Chrysalis* (UK), *Capitol* (US), 2002

The breath is the only thing that is happening *right now*. The Metal element teaches us that when we focus on our breath, we are able to receive the gifts and blessings offered by the present moment. The breathy voice of Scottish singer Angela McCluskey is a classic Metal voice. This upbeat track gets the heart pumping to lift us out of the weight of sadness and reminds us that the best way stay connected to the beauty around us is to breathe … and believe.

"Give Thanks" by India Arie
Album: SongVersation: Medicine, *BMG Rights Management*, 2017

This beautiful, solemn song evokes the power of surrendering our pain, and offering gratitude a higher power for the gift of existence. Gospel greats like "Amazing Grace" and "Peace Be Still," Buddhist chanting, the Sri Lalita Sahasranama, and spiritual songs from every culture and tradition around the world remind us of the transcendent nature of our souls. The Metal element essence helps us to have reverence for life itself—with all its pain and suffering—and to step into the light of divine gratitude. Hallelujah. Amen. Om Shanti. Ase.

Metal in Practice: Create a Release Ritual

The following is a short ritual I use any time I have to let go of someone or something. Just as you can't take back an exhale,[97] I feel a sense of finality and completion when I offer this prayer up to the universe. I set the intention that whatever I inhale next—be it a hobby, habit, friendship, lover, or an opportunity—will be one that brings new life.

When the Metal element is involved, there's an intellectual side of us that often understands what and why we have to let go. But the heart has a whole different experience of grief. I use this ritual to reconcile the two. The Metal element is the last in the cycle and represents a stage of completion. As you'll see, this prayer demonstrates how the Metal element is in a dynamic dance with the other four elements we explored in the previous chapters.

The prayer aspect of the ritual consists of four simple sentiments: Thank you. I love you. I'm sorry. *Asé.*

Step One: Reflection (Metal)

What do you need to let go of? Take a moment to reflect on your experience and decide what has reached a stage of completion and is ready to be exhaled. This might be internal or external—releasing habits or negative thought patterns can be just as powerful as offering this release ritual for a relationship, job, or experience. Once you decide *what* you are going to release, determine *how* you are going to symbolize it. Here are some suggestions:

- Write this prayer in a notebook or journal, followed by shredding or burning the paper when finished.
- Speak this prayer into a candle and then blow out and discard the candle upon completion.

---

97. Erwin Thomas, conversation with author, October 2020.

+ Speak this prayer into a glass water and then pour the water down the drain or into nature (toilet flushes can be immensely satisfying!).
+ Share this prayer with a picture of yourself in childhood or at the time of the wound and close the prayer by bowing deeply to (or having a small party for) your inner child.
+ If appropriate, send this prayer in a letter, text, or email to the person with whom you are seeking completion. However, consider waiting a few days before hitting "send." In many cases, just the act of writing the letter can facilitate an energetic shift; you may not feel a need to share your insights.

Step Two: Thank You (Metal and Earth)

The Earth element teaches us how to have gratitude and guides us as we digest our earthly experiences. The next step in this prayer to us offers gratitude. The Metal element teaches us how to value the preciousness of something and will make us hang on to stuff until we see that value. Though it may seem counterintuitive, the more we are grateful, the easier it is to let go.

What did this person, experience, or thing bring you? How was your life enriched? That's your thank you. It is an expression of why you are grateful, no matter how painful or full of sorrow it may be right now.

Step Three: I Love You (Metal and Fire)

Love connects us to our essence. When people, places, or experiences have come to an end, love remains eternal. Situations of anger, angst, or apathy will continue returning to us, wanting ultimately to become love. What do you love about that which you are now letting go? How can you find the love in this situation or circumstance?

Finding where you can say "I love you" activates the heart of the Fire element. It keeps us from closing up, especially when it's time to move on. However, it is important to find love from an authentic place and to not spiritually bypass yourself by ignoring your own hurts. Your love might be directed to yourself—the growth you've experienced and the qualities you've cultivated. Love might also extend toward the sense of expansion you experience now that you've let go. Finally, offering love to your spiritual source can greatly support the relationship between Metal and Fire.

Step Four: I'm Sorry (Metal and Wood)

The "I'm Sorry" stage of the prayer offers a moment to take responsibility and acknowledge our personal agency, which activates the Wood element. Even in places where we feel like the circumstances were out of our control, saying "I'm sorry" allows us to release guilt and shame while making corrective actions in the future. For example, when my close friend transitioned to the spiritual realm right in the heart of Metal element season, I felt *so* much grief. My "I'm sorry" included "I'm sorry that I did not come hang out as often," and "I'm sorry that I wasn't able to see you one last time." Rather than staying stuck in the shame and self-depreciation, this acknowledgment as part of a release ritual helped me to value and prioritize my living friendships moving forward.

Finding the "I'm Sorry" can be one of the hardest parts of this ritual. Be kind to yourself. And, sorry friends, cynical statements like "I'm sorry you're such an asshole" don't quite work (believe me, I've tried), and tend keep us stuck. Instead, call on the Metal element for support as you reflect on the places where you can internally or externally "do better" without allowing it to take away from your essential worth.

Step Five: Asé (Metal and Water)

Asé (pronounced Ah-SHAY) doesn't have an exact English equivalent. It means that everything is exactly as it is meant to be. It affirms that all is well and is as destined. In this prayer, Asé is the final release and summons the power of the Water element. As you may remember, the Water element offers wisdom through experience and holds the key to divine timing. It reminds us of our destiny. When we say Asé, we accept and surrender to a higher power. We trust that even though we may not have the answers or fully understand, there is an intrinsic order to our lives.

Step Six: Completion

Close the ritual with physical action: shred your paper, blow out your candle, flush your water, or bow to your inner child. As with all soul medicine practices, this release ritual can unfold over several hours, or take just a few minutes in your mind. Trust yourself, and use your intuition to determine the best way to find closure and move forward.

The Metal element teaches us how to surrender, release, and let go so that we can make space for something new. Metal invites us to get rid of clutter, get rid of negative thoughts, get rid of bad habits, and get rid of unhealthy relationships. Metal is the death that makes space for life.

★★★

I met Sheridan more than five years ago. She came into my office on an autumn wind a few short months after her husband drowned in a tragic accident during their summer vacation. Sheridan returned from that family vacation with their two grieving children but without the love of her life.

The grief in the room was palpable. For the first few weeks, Sheridan did not speak much but simply allowed her tears to flow on the treatment table. It was a safe space for her to break down and release in the way that she could not in the presence of her children. She was holding it together in every sense—managing not only her children and her career but also the conflict that emerged from her late husband's family.

Even through her deep sadness and loss, I could see the gifts of the Metal element very early in our process. Sheridan constantly sought the deeper meaning and purpose of her experience. Moving beyond her religious upbringing, she began to study astrology, numerology, and other mystical arts in earnest that could offer some solace and insight into the Great Mystery.

The key signature of the Metal element I experienced with Sheridan was the deep awe, respect, and inspiration I felt in her presence. On many levels it felt selfish—she was coming to me for treatment, yet I was the one getting healed! In everything Sheridan spoke, she transmitted her deep respect and reverence for the spiritual realm. She willed herself to live in the present moment, as her experience had taught her not to take a single second for granted. Her words flowed with the wisdom of someone who knew the trials of the heart the precious gift of life.

Sheridan shared with me a poem that she had written as part of her healing journey. With her permission, I share an adaptation of her original work with you as a beautiful tribute to the Metal element:

I know we all came here to evolve mentally, emotionally, spiritually and physically through the seasons and cycles in our lives.

I know in order to truly evolve, one must put the work in while faithfully walking in our own Presence, and synchronizing with the universe for supernatural guidance and inspiration.

I know life-changing events HAVE to and WILL occur in all our lives to provide us with the opportunities to realign with our Divine path and purpose in order to complete what has already been written in the Stars.

I know we all came here to be the very best version of ourselves, and can evolve through the power of love by having an open heart, mind and spirit, and a willingness to do the required work.

I know my husband's transition was *the* life-changing opportunity in this lifetime that is now giving me the chance to realign myself with my Divine path and purpose.It has reconnected me to my Inner-Divinity and the Divine Feminine all through my journey of grief.

I am choosing to rock with it and live faithfully in the Now because **I know.**

★★★

The Metal element is the last of the elements and represents completion. Yet, just as a circle has no ending or beginning, the journey of the soul is also not a straight line. It is filled with ups and downs, successes and regressions. It feels spiral in nature as we suddenly and unexpectedly find ourselves revisiting wounds that we thought we had healed, and rediscovering gifts we thought we had lost. Metal teaches us that every exhale is followed by an inhale, and every end is followed by a new beginning. We plant a new spirit seed.

Conclusion

"One cannot love his neighbor unless he is aware of his neighbor.
We hope through the understanding of each other's culture that peace
and global harmony will come to mankind; so that we can protect
the only home we have ever known, the plant Earth."
—*Baba Kwame Ishangi*

Osun is an African goddess often depicted carrying a mirror. To deepen my relationship with this goddess as part of my healing, I was introduced to Iya Omiyemi, a priest in the Ifa tradition, to start a spiritual process called Mirror Work. Being the ambitions and super intellectual student I am, I immediately went on Google to look up everything I could find about Mirror Work and added an elaborate gold mirror to my Amazon shopping cart. I prepared for a month or so of gazing at myself in the mirror while reciting positive affirmations in the form of hip-hop lyrics, like Issa Dee on the HBO show *Insecure*.

Iya Omiyemi asked me a single question that stopped me in my tracks: *Where do I go to find a reflection of myself in nature?* The question made me first want to weep. Living in Brooklyn, I felt so disconnected from nature. It had been a long, hard winter. The COVID-19 pandemic shook the world and made "outside" one of the riskiest, most dangerous places to be. The trifecta of the increase in crime, increased police presence in my neighborhood, and increased visibility of police brutality in the media made me stiffen every time I walked out of my door. I felt the tension in my environment in every cell of my being.

I also had to laugh at the incredible irony. Here I was, writing a book about nature and how to recognize its pulse inside of our psyche, yet I wasn't actually taking the time to connect and immerse myself in nature. No wonder I was feeling so blocked!

Iya Omiyemi sent me on a quest to discover my reflection in the natural world. I immediately heard an inner voice tell me to go to the forest. I recalled a whitewater rafting adventure I had gone on in the summer of 2020. During that seventeen-mile wild ride down the Hudson, we encountered a part of the forest that could only be reached by raft. You couldn't drive there for sure, and precious few people would venture to camp in an area that was so untamed and unpredictable. Let me tell you, there is nothing like experiencing nature in full force, undisturbed. I could feel nature's majesty and magic. In the presence of that forest, I felt insignificant in the most wonderful way, full of the humility that we experience in the presence of the Divine.

That was the forest experience I was craving when I decided to venture to Forest Park in Queens. I had often passed the park from the Jackie Robinson Parkway in my comings and goings and had been meaning to go there for some time. I figured that the way it popped up in my mind's eye was surely a sign, so I registered for a group hike through Forest Park the following Sunday. Unfortunately, the majority of the hike took place alongside the parkway, an inside view of what I saw when I drove by in my car. Instead of feeling renewed and recharged, I felt…sad. It was early in the spring and so the leaves were barely budding. Every now and then, a runner on the trail would whiz by, cursing our group for blocking their path. Plus, the steady whoosh of cars in the background were a constant reminder that I was still in the city. This was not the reflection in nature I was craving..

Determined, I next went to the Brooklyn Botanic Garden. Now this, I thought, was the experience I was looking for! I could feel the love and care that had been put into cultivating this magnificent garden. Not to mention that I could see the volunteer workers with their pails of dirt and compost and whatnot lovingly preparing the garden beds for the new season. There were lots of folks strolling around the garden, appreciating and paying attention. They took selfies with the glorious magnolias fresh in bloom. They contemplated alongside the lotus flowers. They rested against the large cherry blossom trees that lined the pavilion. I could feel the flowers appreciating that attention! The garden felt alive and vibrant, and I felt at peace.

Here's the thing: both the Botanic Garden *and* Forest Park are my reflections. When I went to Forest Park, I was devitalized, much like the trees who were navigating the air pollution from the nearby highway. I also felt unseen and taken advantage of in many of my relationships. This was just as I imagined the trees feeling when runners came to the park for solitude and calm, but never stopped to pick up the trash on their path. And just like those early spring trees, there was new life stirring in me that was not yet visible. The imbalance I felt at Forest Park was a reflection of my own imbalance. And in the Botanic Garden, I witnessed the part of my beautiful self that thrives with loving attention and care. I am also a carefully curated garden of magnificence.

Nature is always our mirror, and we are in a reciprocal relationship with the entire universe. A student of Ifa is called an *aborisa*, one who studies self and nature. We learn that to the African mind, reality is phenomenological. This means that our experience, our consciousness, and our interpretation of reality are interdependent. What we notice and what enters our consciousness has meaning. The universe, as nature, is constantly communicating messages to us. This is why an orb weaver spider appeared for my client as she strategized her new business, teaching her about the value of meticulous planning with the expectation of abundance. This is why Forest Park reminded me to build my vitality and the Botanic Garden reminded me that I am loved.

Through working with the five elements and the nature medicine in this book, we can learn to see ourselves as part of the greater cycles, patterns, and mysteries of nature. It is a way that we can reengage with ancestral wisdom; a time when the human body, mind, nature, and spirit were all considered an interconnected whole. African botanist Maurice M. Iwu explains that in most African communities:

> … living is a religious act; healing therefore includes rituals, incantations, and medicines that will remedy both the diseased body and the sick spirit … It is the healer's duty to ensure a symmetrical relationship between his or her patient and the natural world.[98]

Nature is our mirror. In the Old World, every animate or inanimate object in the natural world has a spirit that represents its essence—plants, forests, rocks, streams, and of course, flowers all have intelligence and consciousness.

Can we go back to the past? Nope! Most of us—self included—enjoy too many of the comforts of high-tech society. I try to imagine what my life would

---

98. Maurice M. Iwu, *Handbook of African Medicinal Plants* (New York: CRC Press, 2014), 367.

look like if I had to rise and set with the sun, carve this book on the back of a turtle shell, cook all of my food by open fire, or walk the two-hundred miles between Brooklyn and my closest relative. No thanks! We live in a new world, and membership has its privileges. But can we integrate ancient ways of living in harmony with nature for a healthier, fuller life? Absolutely! Especially now, as social scientists are beginning to understand how our separation from nature is connected to growing anxiety, depression, lack of purpose, and a decreased sense of self and community.[99]

Today, the World Health Organization estimates that more than three-hundred million people worldwide suffer from depression, making it the leading cause of disability.[100] According to the Anxiety and Depression Association of America, nearly one-half of those diagnosed with depression are also diagnosed with an anxiety disorder, which affects forty million adults in the United States age eighteen and older every year.[101]

How did we get here?

We can trace modern psychology's origins to seventeenth-century philosopher René Descartes, best known for his theory of dualism in which he declared the mind and body are two separate, distinct entities. Dualism not only separated the body from the mind, it also separated humans from nature, nature from spirit, and by extension, humans from the spirit of nature. I don't know why everyone took Descartes's word for it, but they drank the Kool-Aid. His idea that the soul is separate from the body laid the foundation for the medicine we know today, one in which the body is seen as a machine with parts that can be studied and treated independently. Specializations within medicine followed soon after, such as obstetrics and gynecology for women's health, cardiology for the heart, pulmonology for respiratory health, and so

---

99. Sofia Softas-Nall and William Douglas Woody, "The Loss of Human Connection to Nature: Revitalizing Selfhood and Meaning in Life through the Ideas of Rollo May," *Ecopsychology* 9, no. 4 (2017): 241–252.

100. Brandi Koskie, "Depression: Facts, Statistics, and You," Healthline (Healthline Media, June 3, 2020), https://www.healthline.com/health/depression/facts-statistics-infographic.

101. "Facts & Statistics: Anxiety and Depression Association of America, ADAA." Facts & Statistics: Anxiety and Depression Association of America, ADAA. n.d., https://adaa.org/about-adaa/press-room/facts-statistics.

on. Matters of the spirit were separated from medicine and placed solidly into the realm of religion. Matters of the mind, including emotions and thoughts, were to be dealt with through psychology.

Then things got really funky. Scientists such as Francis Bacon, inventor of the scientific method, further solidified the worldview that the only reality that exists is the one we can observe and measure. Bacon has gone on the record for saying, "It is important to use techniques of the Inquisition to tease and torture the secrets of Mother nature out into the open."[102] I mean—ouch! This statement ripples through my nervous system, recognizing it as one that has caused much harm to Earth and her people. This perspective also included the beliefs that:

- nature is composed of inert, physical elements;
- these physical elements can and should be controlled; and
- individual human beings seeking private economic gain should control them.[103]

Psychology emerged as a formal field of medicine in the nineteenth century, during the so-called Age of Enlightenment in the Western world. Yet, this age also represents a period of destruction and annihilation of Indigenous people, culture, and land. Nature was no longer perceived as dynamic, alive, or sacred, but rather as another resource to be manipulated as a cog in the great wheel of human civilization.

As the Industrial Revolution flourished, spiritual goals were replaced by materialistic goals, in so much that physical well-being and worldly possessions became the greatest good and the highest value in life. Humanity in the Western world reconsidered its place and purpose. Instead of looking to the heavens, nature, and community for self-definition, people began to look within *themselves*. The Industrial Age brought members out of their homes and families and into the workplace.

---

102. Pam Montgomery, *Plant Spirit Healing: A Guide to Working with Plant Consciousness* (Rochester, VT: Bear & Co., 2008), 12.

103. Susan M. Koger, Winter Deborah Du Nann, and Winter Deborah Du Nann, *The Psychology of Environmental Problems: Psychology for Sustainability* (New York: Psychology Press, 2010), 38.

Today, Western culture continues to celebrate individualism, and places great importance on self-actualization, personal agency, and individual achievement. Some even fear that the "individual is in many ways replacing the family as the basic unit of society,"[104] as evidenced by the higher rates of later marriages, marriages ending in divorce, significantly smaller households, and people moving away from families to explore academic and career goals.[105] This creates a world in which it is easier to accept and strive for independence and to travel our own paths.[106] Though it is changing, modern psychology was designed to help a person achieve personal (individual) success, and to successfully navigate the resources at their disposal.

Unfortunately, this is the lens through which many of us are introduced to nature and plant medicine. We learn about herbs in terms of what they can do for *us*. Herbs featured in clinical case studies and empirical evidence are promoted for our physical symptoms—to clear congestion, boost immunity, or reduce inflammation. Plant medicine and rituals used for their emotional and spiritual impact (including flower essences) are largely discredited as placebos at best and dangerous at worst.

What's missing is from this way of thinking about the mind and the body is the *magic*. We are greater than the sum of our parts, and our bodies are not machines. Our personal success and achievement means little to nothing if we are isolated from everything and everyone. Whether we're talking about organs in the body, people in a party, communities in solidarity, or the flowers in an herbal formula—it's the same truth. The magic is the spirit. We are better together.

A Return: Ecopsychology and the Neo-Ancients

Ecological psycology is an emerging branch of psychology that revisits the principles and philosophies of Indigenous and Diasporic wisdom. Ecopsy-

---

104. Marc Pilisuk and Susan Hillier Parks, *The Healing Web* (Hanover, NH: University Press of New England, 1986). as quoted in Keith J. Karren, N. Lee Smith, and Kathryn J Gordon, *Mind/Body Health: The Effects of Attitudes, Emotions and, Relationships* (Boston: Pearson, 2014), 256.

105. Ibid.

106. Ibid.

chology aims to create a life-celebrating society in which all lives are valued, sacred, and belonging. It reminds us that caring for one another—people and planet—is more important than our individual acheivements. It invites humanity to relearn how to revere and maintain a reciprocal relationship with nature, instead of a relationship of power and dominion. We relearn how to see ourselves as part of the interconnected web of life. In other words, nature is our mirror.

Ecopsychology brings us back what the ancients knew. In his article, *Traditional African Environmental Ethics and Colonial Legacy*, Polycarp A. Ikuenobe describes the ways in which Western colonialism did a number on traditional African spiritual and cultural relationships with nature. He explains that prior to this disruption, "indigenous African societies saw mountains, trees, rivers, and different animals as representations or embodiment of deities and spirits, and as such, they are divine, sacred, and are given due reverence."[107] Now, the environmentalist movement points an accusing finger, offering Ecological Psychology as solution to the environmental problems. It's kind of like if someone stole your sneakers from your gym locker, made fun of you for walking around barefoot, and then sold your sneakers back to you at a price you couldn't afford.

That aside, I love and appreciate ecological psychology because it differs from other forms of psychology in key ways. It's not about connecting to nature purely for self-interest. Though nature can help ease anxiety, depression and boost immunity, the goal of ecological psychology is to support us as we cultivate a harmonious, reciprocal relationship between self, the world, and the Sacred. At its essence, ecological psychology is soul medicine.

Ecological psychology also provides a philosophical framework for a soul squad that I like to call Neo-Ancients. Like the field of ecological psychology, Neo-Ancients live at the intersection of past and future. We honor our magical experiences as much as our logic. And, we enjoy the benefits of modern technology as much as we enjoy the healing offered by ancient traditions. Neo-Ancients want to reclaim a bit of the connection to nature—and connection to ourselves—that we've lost. We are reaching back to embrace our

---

107. Polycarp A. Ikuenobe, "Traditional African Environmental Ethics and Colonial Legacy," *International Journal of Philosophy and Theology (IJPT)* 2, no. 4 (2014): 5.

ancestral beliefs about the web of life. And we are turning to nature's medicine for healing.

Some Neo-Ancients practice yoga. Some get acupuncture. Some walk with essential oils and sprays in our purse just in case someone pisses us off in a work meeting. Some read monthly horoscopes on mainstream websites, while others have an astrologer on speed dial for those particularly tough periods. Some dedicate our lives to traditional practices in earnest while using phone apps that alert us when full moons and Mercury retrogrades are coming. Some of us use CBD-infused gummies or products without ever realizing that we are engaging with plant intelligence. Some are loud and proud of our Neo-Ancient quirkiness, and some enjoy a decidedly more private Neo-Ancient existence by simply incorporating mindfulness into our morning commute. We are everywhere. In our own ways, we realize that our sense of well-being and contentment is as important as our physical health and material success. We seek out the deeper purpose and meaning of our experiences. Neo-Ancients also intuitively know that ancient practices—whether we recognize them as such or not—are an integral part of the future we are co-creating.

Anima Mundi: The Soul of the World

Ecopsychology draws us away from the mind-body split, and instead embraces an ancient concept popularized in classical Greek thought: the *anima mundi,* translated from Latin as the "soul of the world." Rather than placing humans as the height of intelligence, the anima mundi refers to the consciousness and intelligence of the natural world. We are part of the soul of the world. As renowned ecological philosopher David Abram aptly describes:

> Intelligence is no longer ours alone but is a property of the earth; we are in it, of it, immersed in its depths. And indeed each terrain, each ecology, seems to have its own particular intelligence, its own unique vernacular of soil and leaf and sky.[108]

---

108. David Abram, *The Spell of the Sensuous: Perception and Language in a More-than-Human World* (New York: Vintage Books, 2017) as quoted in Andy Fisher, *Radical Ecopsychology: Psychology in the Service of Life* (State University of New York Press, 2013), 12.

Rather than humanity *versus* nature, we experience our humanity *as* nature, placing the human psyche within the psyche of the earth.

Have you ever walked through the woods, and felt something watching you? I experienced this during my yoga teacher training in Costa Rica. At first, I thought it was a bird or squirrel anxiously watching me and ready to bolt at my sudden, crude movements. In scarier moments, I imagined myself being stalked by a large predator, ready to take advantage of my ignorance. I walked slowly and cautiously, sensing something sensing me.

After a long while I realized that there was no jungle cat or scared rodent— it was Earth herself! The leaves in the trees, the bush, the soil, the wildflowers—they all sensed my movement and regarded me with as much intensity as anyone I've ever known. Earth is Gaia, living and breathing. I can't help but think, as I walk through the woods or through a field, that I am walking on the brain of the earth. I imagine the sponginess beneath my feet as the plant world's large, responsive nervous system. It fills me with awe.

Flower Essence Society co-founder Patricia Kaminski explains that the anima mundi is not based on a romantic, sentimental projection, or nostalgia for a mythic golden age.[109] The anima mundi is with us, right here and right now. Like our predecessors, Neo-Ancients also learn how to recognize the archetypal forces of nature as qualities of the human soul. I think of the consciousness of the ocean, I watch her waves ebb and flow. I envision her bringing me blessings with her tide, and washing my worries out to sea. I let the music of her rolling waves lull me to sleep, where I envision myself in the primordial, nurturing womb waters of Yemoja. I also see the ocean's force personified in the Disney movie *Moana*, in which the ocean is a character that guides, nurtures, and supports the heroine on her journey. This is the anima mundi. When we see ourselves in the forces of nature, and see the forces of nature unfolding within ourselves, we share the anima mundi.

Nature is our mirror. Each flower essence in this book is an archetypal mirror of an aspect of the human psyche. We can learn to recognize the five elements as the seasons of our souls. And also, we can sit in a park. Speak to

---

109. Patricia Kaminski and Richard Katz, *Flower Essence Repertory: A Comprehensive Guide to North American and English Flower Essences for Emotional and Spiritual Well-Being* (Nevada City, CA: Flower Essence Society, 2004), 26.

the wind. Listen to the waves. This is how we begin to find our way back. If we can humble ourselves and pay attention, we can reenter a reciprocal relationship with the natural world.

Ecotherapy: Principles in Practice

Ecotherapy—the practice of spending time in nature for personal or spiritual healing—is a growing trend. At one end of the spectrum, ecotherapy is as accessible as buying a plant or spending time outdoors. At the other end of the spectrum, there are elaborate systems to guide clients as they awaken the archetypes of the anima mundi in the human soul. I consider ecotherapy as three layers of practice:

DIY Practices	Communal Practices	Clinical Practices
Spending time in nature	Community Gardening	Acupuncture
Visiting parks	Farming	Astrology
Gardening	Tree-Planting	Flower Essence
Growing Food/Herbs	Composting/Recycling	Therapy
Hiking	Wilderness/Nature Immersions	Herbalism
Indoor Plants	Environmental Justice/Advocacy	Nature Rituals
Camping	Volunteering in an Animal Shelter	Dream Tending
Having Pets		Shadow Work
Mindful Consumption		

DIY Practices

We can all find a way to connect with nature, no matter where we live. Nature is everywhere! We have the creative freedom to design our time with nature in accordance to our preferences, budget, and lifestyle. When I asked the students in my practitioner training program how they connect to nature, they said:

- Gardening and even cutting the tiny lawn connects me
- Walks at the park, gardening, and flower arranging
- I stand in a parking lot and feel the breeze and the sun's kiss
- Listening to rain, dancing in rain, and sitting by rivers, lakes, and beaches
- Running barefoot in the grass, feeling grounded and at peace in the earth

* Following the cycles of the moon in ritual and in ceremony
* Eating super seasonal foods
* Watching the horizon
* Gifting something to the river
* Biking in the magic hour sun with the wind in my hair
* Observing nature, how things come and go, the ways plants move, breathe, and reach out
* Sometimes even just sitting in the grass and staring off at the sky, and remembering we all share this planet
* I love to connect to nature through surrender[110]

One of my favorite ways to connect to nature is through my Mindful Consumption practices, which involves tracing what I purchase back to its natural source as a reminder that everything that exists comes from the earth. I bring this empathetic contemplation to my last meal, a burrito from a local restaurant. It had simple ingredients: corn, beans, cheese, and a tortilla. But when I consider the amount of time, energy, and resources that went into that meal, it's humbling! Can I picture the cow being milked as well as the resources needed to keep that cow fed? Who harvested the corn and wheat, and can I even picture how a black bean grows? As I deepen my reflection, I realize the gaps in my knowledge—the burrito is wrapped in aluminum foil, but how the heck is *that* made? Who packaged the ingredients? What's the ink printed on the brown paper bag made of? How many trees went into making the bag? Where and how were they processed? This simple reflection can go on infinitely, highlighting the ways I personally take the earth for granted.

There are limitless possibilities in which we can experience nature with varying degrees of impact, from deep immersive experiences to simply opening a window or gazing at a natural environment.[111] We can all find a way to integrate nature's healing gifts into our personal lives.

---

110. Students of "Nature Knows: Ecological Consciousness and Reciprocity" (class) Spring 2021, www.TheSpiritSeed.org.

111. Roly Russell et al., "Humans and Nature: How Knowing and Experiencing Nature Affect Well-Being," *Annual Review of Environment and Resources* 38, no. 1 (2013): 473–502.

Communal Practices

Communal practices help us experience ourselves as part of the human family, and honor our reciprocal relationship with nature. They depend on shared knowledge, skills, and collaboration in order to reach a shared goal, which is to leave our world better than we found it. They also cultivate our ability to form healthy and lasting bonds with others with empathy, care, and concern. Communal practices help us to relearn what ecologist Andrew Fisher calls the human art of revering, giving back to, and maintaining reciprocal relationships with the animate natural world."[112] We can play an active role in shaping and building practices that protect and support the environment. This may also include engaging in embodied activism that addresses the many social and environmental issues of concern in the twenty-first century.

Sometimes when we hear words like "environmentalism" and "ecology" we think it refers to something "over there"; there's cognitive dissonance. Now, I'll be the first to admit that there *is* often a disconnect between the fight for the environment, and the fight for human rights. Environmental activist Carl Anthony asks the question that sums up this quandary: "Why is it so easy for these people to think like mountains and not to think like people of colour?"[113] The media doesn't help by creating stereotypical images of granola-eating, radical environmentalists who denounce modern comforts. Television sitcoms are rich with caricatures of nature lovers who hug trees and talk to crystals (I do both). The media tends to present those who care about and advocate for the environment as kooky mystics. But a yes/and instead of an either/or mindset helps break out of that funky mental trap. We can connect to nature, support the environment, *and* live a modern life. We can care for the planet *and* its people. I say yes to all of it.

I have a tremendous amount of awe and respect for those who dedicate their lives to defending the planet, farming the land, and living almost exclu-

---

112. Andy Fisher, *Radical Ecopsychology: Psychology in the Service of Life* (State University of New York Press, 2013), 26.

113. Carl Anthony, "Ecopsychology and the Deconstruction of Whiteness," in *Ecopsychology: Restoring the Earth, Healing the Mind* ed. Theodore Roszak and Mary E. Gomes (San Francisco: Sierra Club Books, 1995), 263–278.

sively off of sustainable materials. I sometimes envision myself living aside a mountain lake in an HGTV binge-inspired tiny house with a compostable toilet. Maybe one day that will be my reality. But until then, I can take simple steps like picking up trash when I see it, recycling, and being mindful of my carbon footprint. For example, I was surprised at how easy it was to start composting. I simply bought a kitchen composting pail for my food scraps. A quick internet search told me what could be composted (coffee grinds, tea, fruit and vegetable scraps) and what couldn't (eggs, meat, dairy products). It was easy (and good exercise!) to walk to the community garden two blocks away to deliver my bag of scraps. And as I considered how the earth composts some waste into fertile soil while other waste rots, I began to make healthier dietary choices. The reciprocity is real: what we do to the earth, we do to ourselves.

Clinical Practices

The relationship between human nature and the intelligence of the natural world is not just poetic—it has practical implications in the field of mind-body medicine. I absolutely love training therapists, acupuncturists, energy workers, and health professionals on the five elements and plant medicine, two of the many ways we can connect our patients to the anima mundi. Many Indigenous and Diasporic nature-based models of soul and soma are still alive today, allowing us to gain incredible wisdom from these ancestral lineages. Flower essences (including the ones you've learned in this book) can be integrated with therapy, herbal medicine, acupuncture, astrology, and spiritual counseling to connect our soul journey to nature's intelligence.

It is so important for us to have a relationship with nature. And it is more important to remember: we *are* nature. The word "human" comes from the Latin *humus*, meaning soil or earth. We are literally made of the stuff of the earth; the same carbon and hydrogen molecules that make up the trees, the grass, and the flowers is the same stuff that makes up our flesh and bones. We are 75 percent water, just like the earth is 75 percent water. The branches of a tree look exactly like the branches of the lungs. Systems of roots—the nervous system of the plant kingdom—look exactly like the network of nerves in our brains. Our veins map our body just as do the rivers streaming to the ocean. Our heart pulses with a sacred rhythm of Earth's heartbeat. The electromagnetic pulse that changes the seasons is the same electromagnetic pulse that changes our psyche. We are of shared pulse, blood, breath, and roots.

At this critical time in the world, we are invited to expand our awareness. We are remembering that the gift of nature healing was once available to all, and passed down for generations like old recipes and folk tales. We are remembering how to listen to nature and honor our intuition. We are paying attention to our deepest desires. We are facing our fears. We are leaning on one another. We are agents of change. We are the ones we've been waiting for.

As the world as we know it transforms before our eyes, the five elements help us tap into our greatest potential.

Nature is our mirror. Go outside and see yourself.

Resources

Where to Find Flower Essences

There are many flower essence companies and practitioners throughout the world. The author encourages readers to explore and contribute to the growing body of flower essence research and experience.

Elementals Flower Essences

Archetypal flower essence formulas created by the author, inspired by the five elements. Each of the formulas are closely aligned with the Soul Lessons explored in this book.
www.ElementalsEssences.com

Flower Essences Services

www.fesflowers.com

Alaskan Essences

www.AlaskanEssences.com

Akika Flower Essences

www.akikafloweressences.com

Classes and Online Education

The Spirit Seed

Professional and personal development flower essence classes offered by the author, including links to playlists and other materials mentioned in this book.
www.theSpiritSeed.org

A New Possibility
Alchemy, Astrology, and Chinese Medicine courses
www.anewpossibility.com

MINKA School of the Healing Arts & Sciences
Wellness and social justice
www.minkamysteryschool.com

The Flower Essence Society
Flower Essence education and research
www.flowersociety.com.

Find a Practitioner

The following sites offer virtual healing services or a directory of local practitioners.

The Spirit Seed
www.theSpiritSeed.org

Black Acupuncturist Association
www.blackacupcunturist.org

MINKA Brooklyn
www.minkabrooklyn.com

Maha Rose
www.maharose.com

The Flower Essence Society Practitioner Referral Network
http://www.flowersociety.org/Practitioner/index.php

Bibliography

Abram, David. *The Spell of the Sensuous: Perception and Language in a More-than-Human World.* New York: Vintage Books, 2017.

Akbar, Na'im. *Know Thyself.* Tallahassee, FL: Mind Productions & Associates, 1999.

Bakare, Lanre. "Trevor Noah: 'It's Easier to Be an Angry White Man than an Angry Black Man.'" *The Guardian.* April 2, 2016.

Brown, Brené. *Daring Greatly: How the Courage to Be Vulnerable Transforms the Way We Live, Love, Parent, and Lead.* New York: Penguin Random House Audio Publishing Group, 2017.

Brown, Timothy T., Juulia Partanen, Linh Chuong, Vaughn Villaverde, Ann Chantal Griffin, and Aaron Mendelson. "Discrimination Hurts: The Effect of Discrimination on the Development of Chronic Pain." *Social Science & Medicine* 204 (2018): 1–8. https://doi.org/10.1016/j.socscimed.2018.03.015.

Butler, Octavia E. *Parable of the Sower.* New York: Grand Central Publishing, 2019.

Campbell, Joseph, Bill D. Moyers, and Betty S. Flowers. *The Power of Myth.* Turtleback Books, 2012.

Chapman, Gary D., and Amy Summers. *The Five Love Languages: How to Express Heartfelt Commitment to Your Mate.* Nashville, TN: LifeWay Press, 2010.

Cheng, Susan. "Apparently, Beyoncé Did the 'Mi Gente' Remix Because of Blue Ivy." BuzzFeed News, October 10, 2017. https://www.buzzfeednews.com/article/susancheng/beyonce-mi-gente-remix.

Dechar, Lorie. *Five Spirits: Alchemical Acupuncture for Psychological and Spiritual Healing*. Asheville, NC: Chiron Publications/Lantern Books, 2006.

Dechar, Lorie Eve and Benjamin Fox. *The Alchemy of Inner Work: A Guide for Turning Illness and Suffering into True Health and Well-Being*. Newburyport, MA: Weiser Books, 2021.

DeGruy-Leary, Joy and Randall Robinson. *Post Traumatic Slave Syndrome: America's Legacy of Enduring Injury and Healing*. Portland, OR: Joy DeGruy Publications, 2018.

"Depression." National Institute of Mental Health website. Accessed September 20, 2021. https://www.nimh.nih.gov/health/publications /depression/index.shtml.

DiAngelo, Robin J. *White Fragility: Why It's So Hard for White People to Talk about Racism*. Boston: Beacon Press, 2020.

Dispenza, Joe. *You Are the Placebo: Making Your Mind Matter*. Carlsbad, CA: Hay House, 2015.

Emoto, Masaru. *The Miracle of Water*. New York: Atria, 2011.

"Facts & Statistics: Anxiety and Depression Association of America, ADAA." ADAA website: https://adaa.org/understanding-anxiety /facts-statistics.

Fisher, Andy. *Radical Ecopsychology: Psychology in the Service of Life*. State University of New York Press, 2013.

"Flower Essence Society: Research, Education, Networking for Mind-Body Health." Flower Society website. Accessed September 19, 2021. http:// www.flowersociety.org/.

Frankel, Lois. *Nice Girls Don't Get the Corner Office: Unconscious Mistakes Women Make That Sabotage Their Careers*. New York: Grand Central Publishing, 2014.

García, Héctor, Francesc Miralles, and Heather Cleary. *Ikigai: The Japanese Secret to a Long and Happy Life*. New York: Penguin Books, 2017.

Gorman, Amanda. *The Hill We Climb: Poems*. New York: Viking Children's Books, 2021.

Gumbs, Alexis Pauline. *Undrowned Black Feminist Lessons from Marine Mammals*. Chico, CA: AK Press, 2020.

Hartman, Eviana. "Are Flower Essences the New Prozac? Inside Fashion's Far-Out Healing Craze." *Vogue*, February 4, 2016.

Hicks, Angela, John Hicks, and Peter Mole. *Five Element Constitutional Acupuncture*. Edinburgh, UK: Churchill Livingstone, 2011.

Hughes, Langston, and Arnold Rampersad. "'Harlem.'" In *The Collected Works of Langston Hughes*. Columbia, MO: University of Missouri Press, 2002.

Ikuenobe, Polycarp A. "Traditional African Environmental Ethics and Colonial Legacy." *International Journal of Philosophy and Theology (IJPT)* 2, no. 4 (2014). https://doi.org/10.15640/ijpt.v2n4a1.

Iwu, Maurice M. *Handbook of African Medicinal Plants*. New York: CRC Press, 2014.

Johnson, Robert A. *Inner Work: Using Dreams and Active Imagination for Personal Growth*. New York: HarperOne, 2009.

Judith, Anodea, and Lion Goodman. *Creating on Purpose: the Spiritual Technology of Manifesting through the Chakras*. Louisville, CO: Sounds True, 2012.

Judith, Anodea. *Wheels of Life: A User's Guide to the Chakra System*. Woodbury, MN: Llewellyn Publications, 2016.

Kaminski, Patricia, and Richard Katz. *Flower Essence Repertory: A Comprehensive Guide to North American and English Flower Essences for Emotional and Spiritual Well-Being*. Nevada City, CA: Flower Essence Society, 2004.

Karren, Keith J., N. Lee Smith, and Kathryn J Gordon. *Mind/Body Health: The Effects of Attitudes, Emotions, and Relationships*. Boston: Pearson, 2014.

Koger, Susan M., and Winter Deborah Du Nann. *The Psychology of Environmental Problems: Psychology for Sustainability*. New York: Psychology Press, 2010.

Koskie, Brandi. "Depression: Facts, Statistics, and You." Healthline website, June 3, 2020. https://www.healthline.com/health/depression/facts -statistics-infographic.

Kumari, Ayele. *The Isese Spirituality Workbook: The Ancestral Wisdom of the Orisa Tradition.* Self-published, 2020.

Larre, Claude, Elisabeth Rochat de la Vallée, and Caroline Root. *The Seven Emotions: Psychology and Health in Ancient China.* London: Monkey Press, 2014.

Lerner, Harriet Goldhor. *The Dance of Anger: A Woman's Guide to Changing the Patterns of Intimate Relationships.* New York: William Morrow & Co., 2014.

"Lilac." Flower Essences Services website. Accessed September 19, 2021. http://store.fesflowers.com/lilac.html.

Linderd. "Lynchings: By State and Race, 1882—1968." *Famous American Trials: The Trial of Sheriff Joseph Shipp, et al.* website. Accessed September 22, 2021: http://law2.umkc.edu/faculty/projects/ftrials/shipp /lynchingsstate.html.

Maciocia, Giovanni. *The Foundations of Chinese Medicine.* Edinburgh, UK: Elsevier Churchill Livingstone, 2005.

Mark, Margaret, and Carol S. Pearson. *The Hero and the Outlaw: Harnessing the Power of Archetypes to Create a Winning Brand.* New York: McGraw-Hill, 2002.

McLaren, Karla. *The Art of Empathy: A Complete Guide to Life's Most Essential Skill.* Louisville, CO: Sounds True, 2013.

Menakem, Resmaa. *My Grandmother's Hands: Racialized Trauma and the Pathway to Mending Our Hearts and Bodies.* New York: Penguin Books, 2021.

Montgomery, Pam. *Plant Spirit Healing: A Guide to Working with Plant Consciousness.* Rochester, VT: Bear & Co., 2008.

Myss, Caroline. *Archetypes: A Beginner's Guide to Your Inner-Net.* Carlsbad, CA: Hay House, 2014.

Ohajunwa, Chioma, and Gubela Mji. "The African Indigenous Lens of Understanding Spirituality: Reflection on Key Emerging Concepts from a Reviewed Literature." *Journal of Religion and Health* 57, no. 6 (2018): 2523–2537. https://doi.org/10.1007/s10943-018-0652-9.

Pennebaker, James W. *Opening Up: The Healing Power of Confiding in Others.* New York: William Morrow & Co., 1990.

Peper, Erik, Annette Booiman, I-Mei Lin, and Richard Harvey. "Increase Strength and Mood with Posture." *Biofeedback* 44, no. 2 (2016): 66–72. https://doi.org/10.5298/1081-5937-44.2.04.

Pilisuk, Marc, and Susan Hillier Parks. *The Healing Web: Social Networks and Human Survival.* Hanover, NH: University Press of New England, 1986.

Redfield, James. *The Celestine Prophecy.* Hoover, AL: Satori Publishing, 1993.

Rhimes, Shonda. *Year of Yes: How to Dance It Out, Stand in the Sun and Be Your Own Person.* Waterville, ME: Thorndike Press, 2016.

Roszak, Theodore, Mary E. Gomes, Allen D. Kanner, and Carl Anthony. "Ecopsychology and the Deconstruction of Whiteness." In *Ecopsychology—Restoring the Earth, Healing the Mind.* San Francisco: Sierra Club Books, 1995.

Russell, James John W. Friedman. *The Grief Recovery Handbook: 20th Anniversary Edition: The Action Program for Moving Beyond Death, Divorce, and Other Losses.* New York: HarperCollins, 2009.

Russell, Roly, Anne D. Guerry, Patricia Balvanera, Rachelle K. Gould, Xavier Basurto, Kai M. A. Chan, Sarah Klain, Jordan Levine, and Jordan Tam. "Humans and Nature: How Knowing and Experiencing Nature Affect Well-Being." *Annual Review of Environment and Resources* 38, no. 1 (2013): 473–502. https://doi.org/10.1146/annurev-environ-012312-110838.

Selassie, Sebene. *You Belong: A Call for Connection.* New York: HarperOne, 2021.

Smith, Rebecca, and Marie Manthey. *Should: How Habits of Language Shape Our Lives.* Minneapolis, MN: Creative Health Care Management, 2016.

Softas-Nall, Sofia, and William Douglas Woody. "The Loss of Human Connection to Nature: Revitalizing Selfhood and Meaning in Life through the Ideas of Rollo May." *Ecopsychology* 9, no. 4 (2017): 241–52. https://doi.org/10.1089/eco.2017.0020.

Somé, Malidoma Patrice. *The Healing Wisdom of Africa: Finding Life Purpose through Nature, Ritual, and Community*. London: Thorsons, 1999.

"Spiritual bypass" Wikipedia. Accessed September 24, 2021: https://en.wikipedia.org/wiki/Spiritual_bypass.

Taylor, Sonya Renee. *Your Body Is Not an Apology: the Power of Radical Self-Love*. Oakland, CA: Berrett-Koehler Publishers, 2018.

"Twelve Windows of Plant Perception." Flower Society website. Accessed September 22, 2021. http://flowersociety.org/twelve.htm.

Washington, Harriet A. *Medical Apartheid: The Dark History of Medical Experimentation on Black Americans from Colonial Times to the Present*. New York: Anchor, 2008.

Wellman, Barry. "*The Healing Web: Social Networks and Human Survival*. Marc Pilisuk , Susan Hillier Parks." *American Journal of Sociology* 93, no. 4 (1988): 1006–1008. https://doi.org/10.1086/228852.

Welwood, John. *Toward a Psychology of Awakening: Buddhism, Psychotherapy, and the Path of Personal and Spiritual Transformation*. Boulder, CO: Shambhala, 2002.

Wilder, Barbara. *Money Is Love: Reconnecting to the Sacred Origins of Money*. London: Cygnus Books, 2010.

Wilheim, Richard, and Cary F. Baynes. *The I Ching or Book of Changes*. Princeton, NJ: Princeton University Press, 1967.

Williams, Justin Michael. *Stay Woke: A Meditation Guide for the Rest of Us*. Louisville, CO: Sounds True, 2020.

Wilson, Vietta E., and Erik Peper. "The Effects of Upright and Slumped Postures on the Recall of Positive and Negative Thoughts." *Applied Psychophysiology and Biofeedback* 29, no. 3 (2004): 189–95. https://doi.org/10.1023/b:apbi.0000039057.32963.34.

Wingfield, Adia Harvey. "The Modern Mammy and the Angry Black Man: African American Professionals' Experiences with Gendered Racism in the Workplace." *Race, Gender & Class* 14, no. 1/2 (2007): 196–212.

Winters, Clyde. *The Ancient Black Civilizations of Asia*, Chicago: Uthman dan Fodio Institute, 2015.

Wohlleben, Peter. *Hidden Life of Trees: What They Feel, How They Communicate*. New York: HarperCollins Publishers, 2020.

Wu, Master Zhongwian. "Daoist Imagery and Internal Alchemy" In *Transformative Imagery: Cultivating the Imagination for Healing, Change and Growth*, ed. Leslie Davenport. London: Jessica Kingsley Publishers, 2016.

Index

This index is divided into three sections to facilitate an easy reference search: general terms, flower essences, and yoga poses.

General Terms

Alchemy, 8, 17, 22, 56, 119, 120, 150, 230, 241, 280

Anger, 7, 38, 39, 49, 72, 81, 83, 84, 86–100, 102, 103, 107, 118, 129, 131, 132, 148, 152, 157, 231, 232, 253, 254, 257, 261

Anima mundi, 272–274, 277

Anxiety, 1, 10, 38, 39, 43, 48, 49, 63, 67, 102, 121, 124, 125, 132, 136, 139, 140, 142–144, 147, 149, 185, 186, 204, 209, 210, 236–239, 268, 271

Astrology, 5, 8, 27, 29, 32, 59, 117, 228, 263, 274, 277, 280

Asé, 124, 260, 262

Attachment, 248, 255

Authenticity/authentic, 1, 41, 43, 71, 103, 111–113, 118, 139, 148, 154, 169, 218, 252, 261

Babalawo, 32

Beauty, 24, 56, 101, 104, 128, 133, 143, 159, 167, 169, 170, 172, 236, 259

Bitterness, 83, 84, 95, 167, 232

Confidence, 43, 85, 110, 114, 117, 123, 127, 138, 171, 178, 242

Deity, 61, 194

Depression, 1, 39, 43, 49, 83, 100, 120, 136, 139, 147, 149, 150, 162, 163, 212, 268, 271

Flower Essence Index

Index of Yoga Asanas

To Write to the Author

If you wish to contact the author or would like more information about this book, please write to the author in care of Llewellyn Worldwide Ltd. and we will forward your request. Both the author and publisher appreciate hearing from you and learning of your enjoyment of this book and how it has helped you. Llewellyn Worldwide Ltd. cannot guarantee that every letter written to the author can be answered, but all will be forwarded. Please write to:

Lindsay Fauntleroy L.Ac.
℅ Llewellyn Worldwide
2143 Wooddale Drive
Woodbury, MN 55125-2989

Please enclose a self-addressed stamped envelope for reply,
or $1.00 to cover costs. If outside the U.S.A., enclose
an international postal reply coupon.

Many of Llewellyn's authors have websites with additional
information and resources. For more information,
please visit our website at http://www.llewellyn.com